ULTIMATE
MILITARY
FITNESS

METRO BOOKS
New York

An Imprint of Sterling Publishing
1166 Avenue of the Americas
New York, NY 10036

Conceived, designed, and produced by
Quid Publishing
Part of The Quarto Group
Level 4 Sheridan House
114 Western Road
Hove BN3 1DD
England

Design and illustration by Rehabdesign

ISBN 978-1-4351-6096-5

For information about custom editions, special sales, and premium and
corporate purchases, please contact Sterling Special Sales at 800-805-5489
or specialsales@sterlingpublishing.com.

Manufactured in China
2 4 6 8 10 9 7 5 3 1
www.sterlingpublishing.com

ULTIMATE MILITARY FITNESS

WORKOUT CHALLENGES OF THE ARMED FORCES

Alexander Stilwell

METRO BOOKS
New York

CONTENTS

INTRODUCTION

In recent years there has been a huge increase in the number of courses available for military style fitness training—and for good reason. People have become aware that military personnel have a level of fitness that allows them to go almost everywhere and do almost anything, not exactly without breaking sweat, but with an ease that is not readily found among those who are either unfit or who specialize in particular sport disciplines.

Military personnel must be able to walk long distances carrying heavy equipment, to climb mountains, to survive for long periods in difficult conditions and, yes, to be ready for anything.

More and more people now aspire to achieving this model of all-round fitness, the closest civilian example of which is cross-training. And what better way to determine whether you meet the military standard than to try some of the tests that recruits have to take to enter military organizations, ranging from the conventional navy, army, and air force intake, to the more specialist requirements of elite and special forces?

Military personnel are not superhuman; they are just people who have set themselves very high standards of fitness as a means to excelling in their chosen military profession.

This book recognizes that a journey begins with a single step; that you need to take stock of where you are and give your body time to adapt to the increased physical activity you will be taking on. It therefore starts with a thorough review

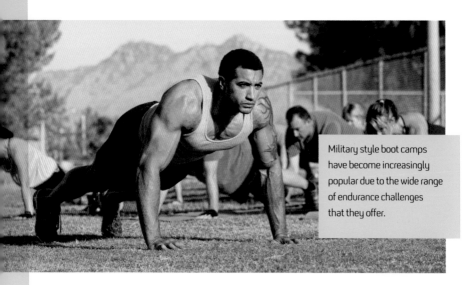

Military style boot camps have become increasingly popular due to the wide range of endurance challenges that they offer.

of your baseline fitness, as well as all of the elements that will contribute to setting you successfully on your journey to fitness. This includes a medical assessment and a thorough review of your diet. As you ask more from your body, you also need to review what you are putting into the tank to make it go. There are helpful tips on finding the right nutritional balance between eating enough to keep you going and not eating too much, so that you lose all those extra unnecessary pounds.

The next part of the book is the military fitness tests themselves. The different tests are described in the context of the national units that set the targets. In this way you will know whether you make the grade as a British Guardsman, US Marine, French Foreign Legionnaire,

or Swedish Special Forces Frogman! Note that the tests are just that—a means of gauging your level of fitness—and should not be used in place of a training program.

In the final part, the individual techniques are explained in more detail, so that you can practice and get yourself in shape in preparation for the specific requirements of each test exercise.

One last thing before we get started: you won't get anywhere without determination and the strength of will to keep going and pick yourself up after the inevitable setbacks. This, ultimately, is what military trainers are looking for. If you follow this journey, you too can achieve ultimate military fitness.

FALL IN

When new recruits arrive at US Marine Corps boot camp, they stand in formation marked out by sets of yellow footprints painted on the ground. This section of the book is about standing in those military footprints and thinking through all the options and challenges that lie ahead. This includes understanding what the tests aim to assess, the range of tests, and what you need to do to clear the bar. Once you have done that, you will be in a much better position to achieve your goals.

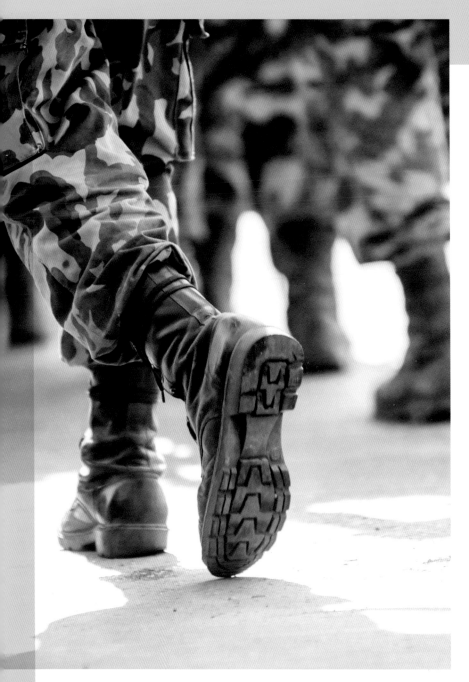

WHY MILITARIES TEST

Military training requires a high standard of both mental and physical commitment and endurance. Military forces need to be confident that they are working with people who have the potential to last the course. By attaining the levels required in the tests, candidates will have already shown that they have some of the qualities that they will need.

Raw Material

Military fitness tests are similar in principle to tests carried out by manufacturing industries on raw materials for their products. While manufacturers invest a great deal of time and money in research and development, military forces and governments invest a great deal of time and money in training and developing raw recruits. By ensuring that the raw recruit meets the minimum standard, there is a far better chance that they will pass through the demanding training program and graduate as effective sailors, soldiers, or air personnel.

Motivation

The military fitness test is not only a test for basic fitness but also for motivation and determination. Those who are able to pass the fitness tests with room to spare have already demonstrated self-motivation by training for the tests. Many military trainers and recruits agree that the real test in military training is the mental test. It is ultimately motivation and the will to succeed that will ensure that a recruit passes successfully through rigorous training.

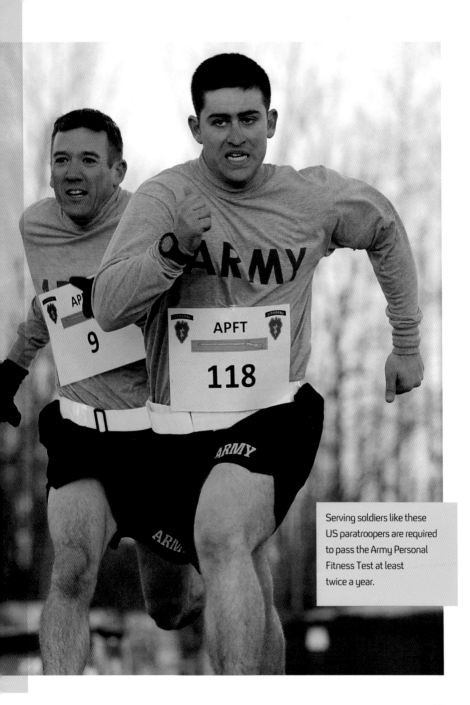

Serving soldiers like these US paratroopers are required to pass the Army Personal Fitness Test at least twice a year.

THE VARIETY OF MILITARY FITNESS TESTS

The recruitment tests run by military forces around the world are in some respects broadly similar, but they do have their own unique aspects and emphasis. The tests can be distinguished by different nations and their traditions but also by the particular roles and types of unit.

The Basics

Across major tests, the basic core tests of push-ups, sit-ups, and a 1.5 or 2-mile (2.4 or 3.2km) run can be found.

The push-up is the most basic and effective exercise for building and testing chest and arm strength using the weight of the body. It is a relatively simple exercise, yet also complex in that it requires a high level of proprioception (the body's mechanism for coordinating movement) to get the technique right (keeping back and legs straight while you touch your chin to the ground).

The sit-up is an effective anterior core exercise that strengthens and conditions the rectus abdominis, or abs.

The pull-up is a very challenging bodyweight exercise that targets the upper back, biceps, and core muscles.

Running is the most basic aerobic exercise and it provides an excellent fitness platform on which to build other exercises.

Military forces are not looking for athletic performance in any one of these disciplines but rather for a snapshot of the recruit's overall physical fitness and aptitude for the broad range of military physical challenges. The underlying concept behind the fitness programs is versatility, because there is no set pattern of activity to prepare for—unlike training for a particular sport, where there is a level of predictability. So the training is effectively cross-training, including aerobic and anaerobic exercise.

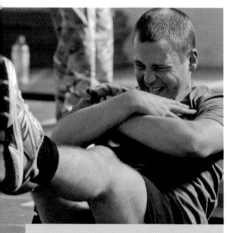

Sit-ups are one of the most regularly used components of fitness assessments. They are a good test of abdominal strength.

Different Approaches

The requirement for versatility and the element of unpredictability has given food for thought to some military sports scientists. The different approaches adopted by units tend to reflect the demands that will be made on recruits once they are out in the field. The current US Army Basic Training Physical Fitness Test consists of the expected mix of push-ups, sit-ups, and a 2-mile (3.2km) run. However, a new test has been proposed that would more accurately test the recruit's strength, endurance, and mobility for typical military scenarios and activities. The proposed test would include a 60yd (55m) shuttle run, to reflect the dash and stop movements that soldiers often have to perform when on a battlefield; a 1-minute rower, which calls for leg and arm coordination; the standing long jump, reflecting the practical military need to negotiate obstacles; and a 1.5-mile (2.4km) run, designed to reflect the more intense running required in battlefield conditions. The new tests are designed to gauge the recruit's anaerobic and aerobic endurance. The intensity of the exercises will show up those recruits who do not have the capacity to keep going under intense stress and muscle fatigue.

> ## ELITE FORCES TEND TO THROW IN ADDITIONAL ELEMENTS TO THEIR TESTING

The British Army have also taken steps to mix it up a bit. The test run by the Army Development and Selection Centre (ADSC) more closely reflects the realities of military life than the sanitized regimes of a gym. Although the test still includes the standard push-ups (minimum of 44 in 2 minutes) and sit-ups (minimum of 50 in 2 minutes), as well as a 1.5-mile (2.4km) run in under 9:30 minutes, there is also a practical static lift of an 88lb (40kg) bag to a height of 4.8ft (1.45m)—and what can be more practical than a jerrican test, where the recruit carries two 44lb (20kg) water containers over a course of 130yd (120m) in under 2 minutes?

The UK Royal Navy choose to test their budding recruits scientifically on a treadmill on which they must complete a 1.5-mile (2.4km) run in under 11:09 minutes for men and 13:10 for women.

They also throw in a shuttle run of 5 × 60yd (55m) and, as it's the Navy, a swimming test. The swim test is reality based and includes jumping into the water in overalls and treading water for 2 minutes before swimming 55yd (50m) to the side and climbing out. These are the sort of skills you will need when abandoning ship.

The UK RAF are among many forces that use the multi-stage fitness test (MSFT) or bleep test in their assessments. This is designed to test progressive aerobic cardiovascular endurance and is also used by coaches for sports such as rugby. The minimum male requirement for RAF entry is a score of 9.10.

Elite Forces

Elite forces tend to throw in additional elements to their testing and raise the bar in areas that are common across most fitness tests. The US Rangers include a 5-mile (8km) run to be completed in under 40 minutes. Recruits who want to enter the Royal Marines All Arms Commando Course (AACC) also need to complete practical tests such as a Fireman's Carry and a rope climb, both done with the correct technique.

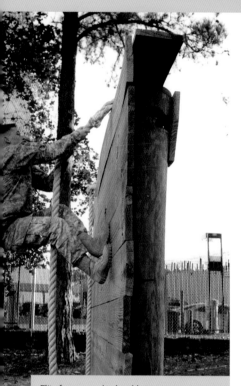

to accompany any special operations unit anywhere in the world, whether by air, land, or sea. Entry tests include 2 × 65yd (20m) underwater as well as a 547yd (500m) swim in under 14 minutes.

To join the Australian Special Forces, recruits need to pass the Special Forces Screen Test where, among other tests, they must achieve a minimum bleep test rating of 10.1, complete a 3-mile (5km) march carrying 88lb (40kg), and pass a swim test that involves treading water for 2 minutes before swimming 437yd (400m) in combat uniform.

Elite forces need to be able to surmount obstacles quickly and efficiently in order to achieve their objectives.

Special Forces

Special forces are required to accomplish a wide range of tasks to a very high standard and their tests reflect this, none more so than the test for entry to the role of US Combat Controller in Air Force Special Operations Command (AFSOC). These specialist operators have to be able

TESTING YOURSELF

The recruitment tests run by military forces around the world are in some respects broadly similar, but they do have their own unique aspects and emphasis. The tests can be distinguished by different nations and their traditions but also by the particular roles and types of unit.

Recreate Realistic Conditions

Most militaries go to great lengths to establish detailed test procedures and conditions, to ensure accurate, reproducible results. If you want to prepare yourself to actually join a particular unit, you might wish to recreate the required test conditions as closely as possible. Much more likely, though, your objective is to challenge yourself against recognized, rigorous standards, so there's no need to go overboard on authenticity: some compromises are okay and in some cases will be necessary.

Environment

Some events, including the bleep test (see page 166), can only be conducted indoors. Others, such as push-ups and sit-ups, can be done either indoors or out, while some running events must be performed outdoors. Most armed forces will not conduct outdoor tests in weather conditions that will significantly affect performance. Many units will not run tests in extreme temperatures, and neither should you.

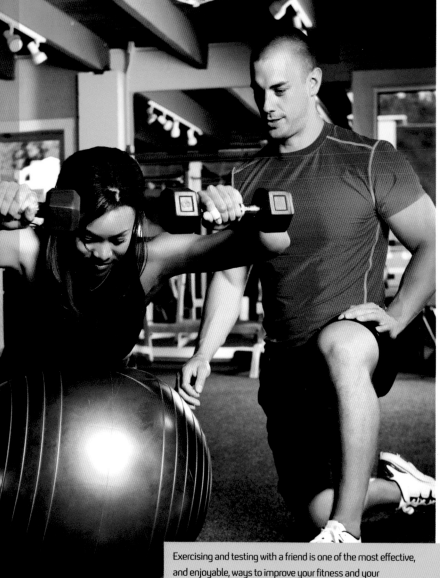

Exercising and testing with a friend is one of the most effective, and enjoyable, ways to improve your fitness and your performance. Friendly competition will spur you both to do your best, and a little peer pressure is a good thing on those days when you're tempted to skip your workout.

USE AN EXERCISE PROGRAM TO GET FIT; USE THE TESTS TO MEASURE YOUR PROGRESS

Equipment

Most events require little in the way of special equipment. A pull-up bar, an exercise mat, a sandbag, and perhaps a stool or box of a certain height will often suffice. Some events, however, are gear-dependent. The Danish Armed Forces use expensive equipment to take direct measurements of VO_2 max during a bicycle ergometer test. You're unlikely to have access to such equipment, but VO_2 max can be extrapolated by indirect methods.

Clothing

Most tests are conducted in conventional exercise clothing: a t-shirt, short pants or sweatpants, and athletic shoes. Purpose-designed running shoes are not the best footwear for events that test agility or require quick changes of direction or frequent stop-starts. For these, more general-purpose exercise shoes are a better choice: they offer superior traction and support in all directions. Some armed forces specify that events be performed in fatigues, and some runs are conducted with full battle gear. You can make do with reasonably similar civilian clothing, boots, backpack, and any carried object of approximately the right weight.

Timing

Most events are timed. Performance may be tested within a fixed time period (for example, the number of sit-ups you can do in exactly 2 minutes), or your time to complete a defined event or task may be measured (for example, how long it takes you to run 5 miles/8km). For events with a fixed time period, you will need a timer with an alarm to tell you when to stop. A stopwatch is needed to time the completion of a fixed task.

Observers

Most events require careful adherence to form and details. For example: your back and legs must remain perfectly straight during a push-up, and your foot must touch or cross the line in the bleep test. Especially if you are new to an exercise, it is helpful to have a friend watch you closely to confirm that you're using proper form and to correct any errors. After you know how to do it right, you'll develop a feel for proper form and may be able to run certain tests without assistance.

Challenging Yourself

There may be a temptation to start at the top and see if you meet the standards of the world's most elite Special Forces units. Resist it. Even among serving infantry, it's a rare individual who can pass those tests, much less avoid hurting themself in the attempt. Start with recruitment or induction tests—the kind that some armed forces administer to determine if you're fit enough to enter basic training. If you can pass those with ease, you're ready to move on to the tests required to pass basic training, or the "in-service" tests that soldiers are required to pass annually. If you fail the recruitment tests, get into a basic fitness training routine and work your way up. At every stage, fitness improves gradually as a result of hard work and consistent, dedicated training. There are no shortcuts, but it's certainly possible to go backward if you work too hard.

Improving Your Performance

Don't confuse fitness testing with exercise. They're different activities, with different objectives. In short: Use an exercise program to get fit; use the tests to measure your progress. There are two ways to improve your performance in an event. The first—employing testing strategies—helps your score a small amount but does not really improve your fitness. Testing strategies are minor things like holding your arms "just so," or deciding at what point during a test to demand the maximum effort.

The other, more meaningful way is long-term training targeted at improving not test performance specifically, but the general type of fitness that the event is designed to assess. So to maximize your performance in (for example) a sit-up event, you'd engage in a broad program of exercises to improve your overall abdominal strength and endurance.

GETTING FIT

The initial fitness tests for military entry are designed to test potential. The instructors do not expect to see the standard of fitness required for more advanced training but they do need to see that recruits have the basic foundations on which to build. Similarly, you can use the military tests in this book in order to gauge your own potential. If you want to improve on your results, you will need to work hard on your strength, stamina, and confidence.

Start Slowly

A journey of a thousand miles begins with a single step. It is a good idea to build your level of fitness up slowly, bearing in mind that your body needs time to change. As you get going with your fitness program, unseen changes take place in your body: your bones become more robust; your joints work more efficiently; the walls of your heart expand and your circulation improves; the number of blood vessels increases and mitochondria in your muscle cells multiply; and fast-twitch muscles in your body increase their resistance to fatigue.

The body responds and adapts in proportion to the strain placed upon it. Increasing fitness is a series of building blocks whereby you place strain on one area of your body and, having given it time to adapt and rebuild, focus on another part.

Mix It Up

Military fitness is all about complete body fitness. There are certain core areas that you need to work on to cover all the bases for military fitness tests: running, upper-body exercises, swimming, and circuit training.

Warm-ups and stretches are a vital component of fitness preparation, both before and after your training session.

Warming up

In order to minimize the risk of injury and also to maximize your performance in a fitness session, you should take time to perform a comprehensive warm-up. During the warm-up, your body temperature is raised and the mobility of your joints is improved through the increased production of synovial fluid. Your muscles are loosened and extended so that they are better prepared to handle a workout.

A warm-up should be done gradually. Your body needs time to transition effectively from a relatively static state to an active one: during this time there is increased blood flow to muscles, airways and blood vessels dilate, oxygen in the blood increases, and there is a reduction in the negative effects of lactic acid and carbon dioxide.

Without a warm-up, there is increased risk of pulling a tendon or muscle or of going into your workout too fast with lungs burning. A warm-up also means that the body will enter the workout with a regular rhythm, whereas without one you often start too fast and quickly taper off.

Suggested warm-ups

1. **To raise the pulse:** Do any of a range of gentle exercises such as jogging, cycling, skipping, or rowing.

2. **Mobility:** Choose from a variety of upper-body mobility exercises, such as arm circles, shoulder shrugs, trunk twists, arm bends, and neck rolls.

3. **Dynamic stretching:** This is designed to increase the flow of lubricating synovial fluid in the joint area and to optimize muscle movement. There are a number of dynamic stretches illustrated on the page opposite. These can be selected according to the particular preferences of the individual and the workout that is to be performed.

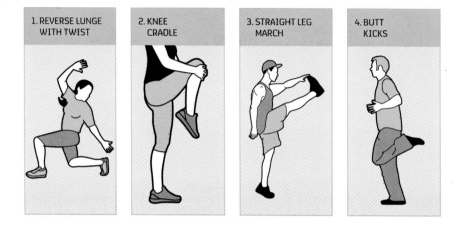

1. REVERSE LUNGE WITH TWIST

2. KNEE CRADLE

3. STRAIGHT LEG MARCH

4. BUTT KICKS

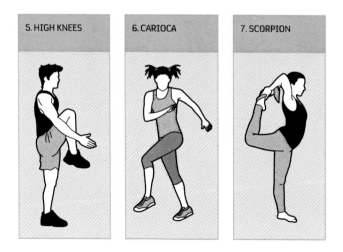

5. HIGH KNEES

6. CARIOCA

7. SCORPION

Post-Workout

The importance of cooling down after exercise is sometimes underestimated. Immediately after exercise your heart is still pumping at a high rate and your blood vessels are dilated. Your limbs, muscles, and joints will also be warm and liable to a build-up of lactic acid. The cooling-down process allows your body to readjust. A short walk of about 5 minutes and static stretching can help prevent your muscles from becoming cramped.

UPPER CALF STRETCH

- Stand 2–3ft (60–90cm) away from a wall with feet flat on the ground
- Lean forward; place your palms on the wall
- Lift your left heel off the ground, keeping your right foot flat
- Keep your knee, hip, and back straight
- Bend your elbows and lean forward
- Feel the stretch in your right calf
- Repeat with the other leg

LOWER CALF STRETCH

ILLIOTIBIAL BAND STRETCH

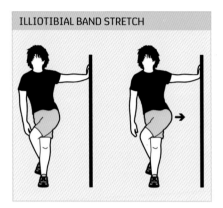

- Stand straight, facing a wall
- Place your palms on the wall
- Bend your left knee and lift your left heel, keeping the right foot flat
- Bend your right knee and lower body
- Feel the stretch at the base of your calf
- Repeat with the other leg

- Stand 2–3ft (60–90cm) away from the wall at right angles
- Cross legs and lean toward wall
- Place the palm of your right hand on the wall
- Keep your right knee and elbow straight
- Push your hips toward wall
- Feel the stretch on outside of left thigh
- Repeat for other thigh

STANDING LAT STRETCH

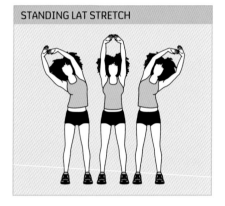

SHIN STRETCH

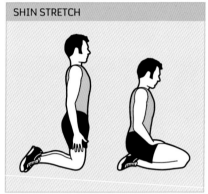

- Grab a handhold with your left hand
- Move your feet back and lean forward
- Keep your upper body parallel to ground
- Your arm should be fully extended
- Lean toward left arm
- Lean back
- Feel the stretch in your lats and shoulder
- Repeat for other side

- Kneel down with your ankles and feet together and toes behind
- Sit down slowly with your heels under your buttocks
- Push your ankles toward the floor
- Keep your ankles together
- Feel the stretch in your shins

GROIN STRETCH

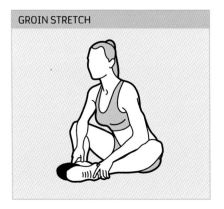

BUTTOCK STRETCH

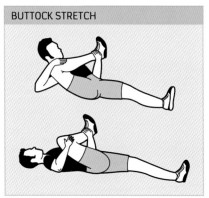

- Sit on the floor
- Pull the soles of your feet together
- Place your hands on your feet
- Rest your elbows against your knees or thighs
- Push your knees toward the floor
- Feel the stretch in your groin

- Lie on your back with your left leg straight
- Bend your right leg back toward your hip
- Rotate your right heel toward your left hip
- Hold your right ankle with your left hand
- Hold your right knee with your right hand
- Pull your leg back toward your shoulders
- Feel the stretch in your right buttock
- Repeat for your left buttock

HAMSTRING STRETCH

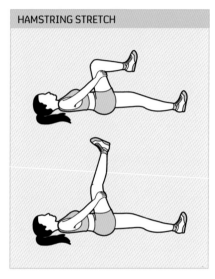

THIGH STRETCH

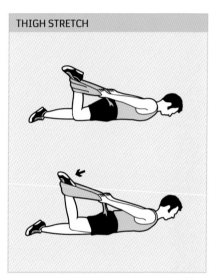

- Lie on your back with your left leg straight
- Bend your right knee
- Bring it back toward your hip
- Grasp your right hamstring
- Straighten your leg
- Feell the stretch in your hamstring
- Repeat for your other hamstring

- Lie on your stomach with your left leg straight
- Bend your right leg at an angle of 90 degrees
- Pass a rope or towel round your right ankle and hold on to both ends
- Raise your right leg off the ground
- Attempt to straighten the knee against the tension of the rope or towel
- Feel the stretch in your thigh
- Repeat for your left thigh

KNEELING HIP FLEXOR STRETCH

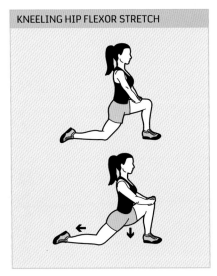

- Kneel on the floor and take a large step forward
- Your front shin should be vertical
- Your rear leg should be stretched behind
- Move your hips down toward the floor
- Slide your leg further back if necessary
- Place your hands on your front thigh and hold the stretch
- Repeat with your other leg

Recovery

After exercise, it is important to refuel your body so that it can enter its recovery phase and so you are ready for action the next day.

- **Replace fluids:** Your body uses a large quantity of water during exercise, especially if you have been out on an endurance run for a long period. Maintain a regular intake of water after exercise and monitor your level of hydration. Keep drinking little and often.
- **Eat within the recovery window:** It makes a big difference to your speed of recovery how soon you eat after finishing exercise. Ideally, you should eat within half an hour, or at most an hour, of the end of your exercise session. To help your body recover quickly, eat a snack with a mixture of complex carbohydrate and protein.
- **Have a shower or bath:** The water will clear your skin pores. Varying the water temperature from warm to cool can also help your blood vessels to clear tissues of waste.
- **Rest:** You have earned it. While you are watching TV or reading a book your body can get on with the process of rebuilding and recovery.

Running

Running is a key way to improve aerobic fitness. This means that your body will be better able to take in and move oxygen around your body. As aerobic fitness improves, your heart and lung capacity increases and your blood system becomes more efficient at transporting oxygenated blood to, and deoxygenated blood away from, your muscles. Aerobic exercise should ideally be performed at between 60 and 90 percent of your maximum heart rate (MHR). Running training can be performed in various ways.

Long slow distance training (LSD)

Running long distances at a steady pace is an excellent base for other types of fitness training as it increases aerobic fitness and builds endurance. It helps to burn fat. However, if you are aiming for the all-round level of fitness required at military standard, take care not to overdo the LSD training. The body of a long-distance runner (often light and lean) is not best placed to perform the full range of demands, such as carrying weights, that a militarily fit person may be required to perform.

Fartlek

Fartlek, from the Swedish, means "speed play." It is a form of interval or speed training that is well suited to the demands of military fitness regimes. It involves alternating fast running with slower jogs. When doing a fartlek run, you may be running at a regular pace, then take long, slow strides for the countdown of a minute, or until you reach a particular marker that you have identified in the distance, such as a tree or lamp post. The training method can also be used in other activities such as swimming.

Fast continuous running (FCR)

This means running at your maximum sustainable pace for an entire run. In other words, it is not the equivalent of a sprint but it means running as fast as you can regularly sustain for the distance you have decided on (which will normally be much shorter than your usual slower rate run distance). This form of running is also an excellent method of burning excess calories. FCR should not be used until you have reached an adequate level of fitness.

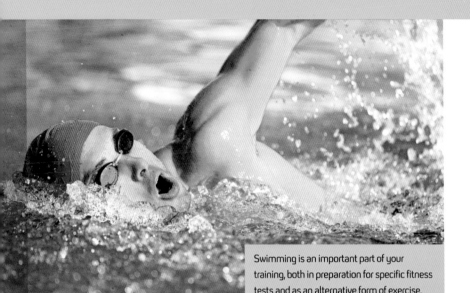

Swimming is an important part of your training, both in preparation for specific fitness tests and as an alternative form of exercise.

Other Aerobic Exercise

Swimming has similar benefits to running in terms of all-over body conditioning. The main difference is that the body is supported by the water and therefore does not have to carry its own weight. Muscles recover more quickly after swimming than after running. It provides a useful alternative to running, allowing your running muscles to recover. Many army physical fitness tests include a test for swimming ability.

Cycling is another good cross-training exercise that complements your running training. While supporting the main weight of the body, cycling allows you to strengthen a number of leg-related muscles, including the gluteal muscles (buttocks), quadriceps (large muscles on the front of the thigh), hamstrings (back of the thigh), and calf muscles.

Rowing helps to build strength and also improves mobility. Despite appearances, rowing places considerably greater emphasis on the legs (70 percent) than on the upper body (30 percent). Efficient rowing, whether in a boat or on a rowing machine, helps you to develop your leg, back, and arm muscles.

Weight Training

Weight training is an important component of your fitness program as it will help to build the core stability and strength that provides a firm platform for other exercises. It will also build the muscles you need to cope with some of the demanding aspects of military fitness testing.

Weight training fits very well with the concept of military fitness because military life involves carrying or moving weights, sometimes over long distances, sometimes requiring short spurts of energy and strength. A soldier, for example, may be required to walk a long distance with all their equipment and then dig a trench.

The strong core muscles built up through weight training help to provide stability for both walking and running, as well as other strength-related activities.

BENCH PRESS

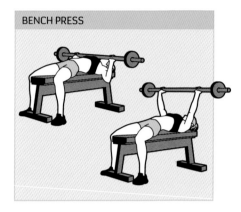

Bench press

Repeat about 20 times, depending on your level of strength and fitness.

- Lie on a bench in a multi-gym or use a manageable barbell
- Shoulders should be directly under the weights
- Place your feet flat on the ground
- Grasp bar or handles
- Push the weight until arms are straight
- Lower slowly again

Shoulder press

You do this exercise either seated or on a multi-gym with support for your back, or it can be performed standing with a barbell. Perform repetitions of 12, depending on your strength and fitness.

- Place hands on the bar slightly under your shoulders
- Hold bar at back of neck
- Slowly push it upward
- Lower slowly to the previous position

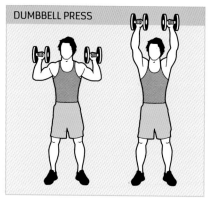

DUMBBELL PRESS

Tricep dip

This exercise works your triceps. Find a sturdy chair, bench, or low wall and sit down on it with your hands by your side and knuckles facing out. Perform 3 sets of 10 repetitions.

- Push legs out in front
- Maintain slight bend in knees
- Use hands for support
- Move buttocks off the bench
- Lower yourself down
- Take the strain in your arms until your elbows are at 90 degrees
- Push back up through your arms until they are straight

Dumbbell press

Try doing sets of 18 repetitions, depending on your strength and fitness.

- Stand with feet shoulder-width apart and your back straight
- Hold a dumbbell just in front of each shoulder
- Raise one above the head and back to its position
- Repeat with the other arm

BENT LATERAL RAISE

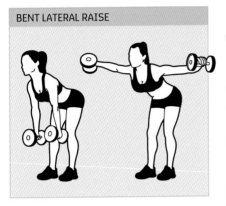

Bent lateral raise

Perform 3 sets of 10 repetitions.

- Bend forward and hold a dumbbell in each hand near your knees
- Raise both arms until straight and more or less parallel with the ground

Lateral raise

Do about 20 repetitions, depending on your level of strength and fitness.

- Lie on a bench with your feet resting flat on the bench and your knees raised
- Hold two dumbbells above your chest, one in each hand
- Keeping elbows bent, lower the dumbbells to the sides then raise them again

Side lateral raise

- With your feet shoulder-width apart and a straight back, hold a dumbbell in each hand by your waist
- Raise both dumbbells simultaneously
- Keep your arms straight
- Slowly lower them to previous position
- Try sets of 12 repetitions, depending on your strength and fitness

Curls

Try to complete 20 repetitions in each set, depending on your strength and fitness.

- Place your feet shoulder-width apart
- Hold either the curling bar from a multi-gym or a barbell at waist level
- Keep your elbows in to your sides
- Curl the bar up to your shoulders and then back down again

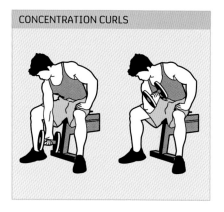

Concentration curls

Try doing sets of 12 repetitions, depending on your strength and fitness.

- Sit on a bench with a dumbbell in your right hand
- Rest your right elbow on your right leg
- Slowly curl the dumbbell up toward your shoulder
- Lower slowly
- Repeat with the other arm

Crunches

Perform 3 sets of 10 repetitions.

- Lie on your back with legs bent and feet flat on the floor
- Place your hands behind or next to your head
- Raise your upper body
- Move both elbows towards both knees

Once you have raised yourself as far as you can, lower yourself to the ground before the next raise. An alternative method is to try to touch the opposite knee each time (e.g., front elbow on left knee).

V-crunches

- Lie on your back
- Place your hands behind your head
- Keep your knees slightly bent
- Lift your upper body
- Also raise your knees
- Touch your elbows to your knees

CRUNCH TECHNIQUE

Try doing abdomen exercises without your legs locked so that your abdominal muscles have to do the work rather than your legs and lower back muscles.

SEATED LEG PUSH

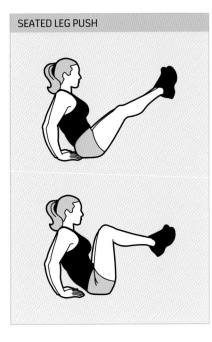

Seated leg push

Do about 30 repetitions in each set, depending on your strength and fitness. Either sit on a bench or on the floor.

- Sit upright supported by your hands
- Raise your legs
- Bring your knees to your chest, then straighten your legs
- Keep your feet off the ground throughout the exercise

Squat

Perform 3 sets of 8 repetitions.

- Stand up straight with your feet shoulder-width apart and your arms folded across your chest
- Bend at the knees, slowly lowering your hips backward and down
- Stop when your thighs are parallel with the floor
- Keep your back straight and push up through your heels back to the starting position

Split squat

This exercise uses hamstring and buttock muscles. Perform 3 sets of 8 repetitions.

- Stand with your feet shoulder-width apart
- Step forward with one foot and back with the other
- Your back foot rests on the toes
- Fold your arms across your chest
- Keep your back straight
- Lower your hips straight down
- Place your weight on the heel of your front foot
- Lower your hips until your front leg is bent at 90 degrees
- Keep your front knee in line with your foot
- Push back up from your heel into the starting position

Step-up

This exercise works your thighs, buttocks, and hamstrings.

- Fold your arms across your chest
- Place one foot on a step or platform (about 16in/40cm high)
- Lean forward slightly
- Move your weight onto the front foot
- Push through the heel of the front foot
- Place your rear foot on the platform
- Slowly step back down to the starting position

Leg raises

Try to do 30 repetitions in each set, depending on your strength and fitness.

- Lie on your back with your hand next to your body or tucked under your buttocks
- Keep your legs straight
- Raise your feet about 6in (15cm) off the ground
- Raise them further to about 20in (50cm) off the ground
- Lower them back down to 6in (15cm)
- Raise them again

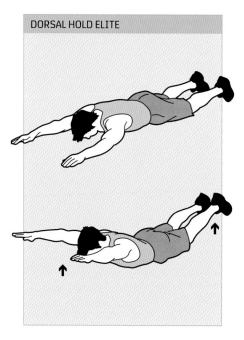

DORSAL HOLD ELITE

Dorsal hold elite

Perform 12–15 repetitions.

- Lie face down on an exercise mat
- Stretch your arms out in front
- Place them on the floor
- Keep your arms and legs straight
- Lift both arms and legs at the same time
- Hold the position for a few moments and then relax back to your original position

FITT TRAINING

The Canadian Armed Forces are aware of the need for their potential recruits to build up their fitness before attempting the entry tests. For this reason they have devised a program called FITT, which stands for Frequency, Intensity, Time, and Type. This is just one approach that you can use to give structure to your training regime.

FITT Guidelines

Frequency: You need to challenge yourself so that your fitness levels increase, while also allowing yourself enough rest for your body to rebuild. Change can sometimes be as good as a rest, so switch between running, cycling, and swimming.

Intensity: As you get fitter, you need to keep increasing the intensity of the exercise to maintain progression. In aerobic exercise you can measure the intensity by using a heart-rate monitor or by running on a treadmill. With strength training you can measure the intensity by the increased workload, which may include bigger weights and more repetitions.

Time: This is an important factor. You need to think about the duration of each workout so that you get the maximum benefit without overdoing it and risking illness or injury. Time can also mean finding the best time for exercise that suits your schedule. Longer workouts are probably best done in the afternoon when your body is warmed up.

> # FITT IS JUST ONE APPROACH THAT YOU CAN USE TO STRUCTURE YOUR TRAINING REGIME

Type: Broadly speaking, the types of exercise are aerobic exercise for cardio fitness and resistance training for muscular strength. Within these categories you can break aerobic exercise down into different types, such as walking, running, swimming, and cycling, and resistance training into the various forms such as push-ups, and barbell and dumbbell training.

When using the FITT guidelines, don't forget a 5–10-minute warm-up and cool-down at the beginning and end of each session. Your main session of strength and aerobic exercise should last between 20 and 60 minutes.

FITT Aerobic session example

Frequency: Three to five times per week, gradually increasing to four or five times.

Intensity: Between 65 and 95 percent of your maximum heart rate.

Time: Begin with exercise sessions of about 20 minutes for the first few weeks and then gradually add on 2 or 3 minutes to each session.

Type: Walk before you run and gradually increase distance, intensity, and variety.

FITT Strength Training

Frequency: Two or three times per week.

Intensity: Lift the appropriate weight the set number of times.

Time: Between 15 and 60 minutes, gradually increasing by 2 or 3 minutes each week.

Type: Ranges from push-ups and sit-ups through to free weights and resistance machines.

AUSTRALIAN DEFENSE FORCE FITNESS PLAN

Many military organizations provide information so that candidates can prepare for the fitness test. This is a good example of a manageable incremental fitness program, which you can adapt to your own schedule and needs.

	Week One	Week Two
Mon	**Morning:** Brisk walk for 30–40 minutes. **Afternoon:** Push-ups. 10 reps. 8 reps. 6 reps. 3 times through. 2 minutes rest between sets. Sit-ups. 10 reps. 8 reps. 6 reps. 3 times through. 2 minutes rest between sets.	**Morning:** Walk for 35–45 minutes. **Afternoon:** Run for 1.1 miles (1.8km).
Tues	**Morning:** Light run for 0.9 miles (1.5km). **Afternoon:** Cycle ride/walk for 30–40 minutes.	**Morning:** Push-ups. 12 reps. 10 reps. 8 reps. 3 times through. 1:45 minutes rest between sets. Sit-ups. 12 reps. 10 reps. 8 reps. 3 times through. 1:45 minutes rest between set. **Afternoon:** Walk for 35–45 minutes.
Wed	Push-up and sit-up routine any time of day (refer to Monday afternoon).	Rest day.
Thurs	**Morning:** Walk for 30–40 minutes.	**Morning:** 35–45-minute cycle ride or walk. **Afternoon:** Push-up and sit-up routine (refer to Tuesday morning).
Fri	Rest day.	Rest day.
Sat	**Morning:** Push-up and sit-up routine (refer to Monday afternoon).	**Morning:** Run for 1.1 miles (1.8km). **Afternoon:** Push-up and sit-up routine (refer to Tuesday morning).
Sun	Rest day.	**Morning:** Walk for 35–45 minutes.

Week Three	Week Four	
Morning: Run for 1.2 miles (2km). **Afternoon:** Push-ups. 14 reps. 12 reps. 10 reps. 3 times through. 1:30 minutes rest between sets. Sit-ups. 14 reps. 12 reps. 10 reps. 3 times through. 1:30 minutes rest between sets.	**Morning:** Walk for 45–55 minutes. **Afternoon:** Push-ups. 16 reps. 14 reps. 12 reps. 3 times through. 1:15 minutes rest between sets. Sit-ups. 14 reps. 12 reps. 10 reps. 3 times through. 1:15 minutes rest between sets.	Mon
Morning: Walk for 40–50 minutes.	**Morning:** Run for 1.4 miles (2.3km). **Afternoon:** Walk for 45–55 minutes.	Tues
Morning: Run for 1.2 miles (2km). **Afternoon:** Push-up and sit-up routine (refer to Monday afternoon).	Rest day.	Wed
Morning: Walk for 40–50 minutes.	**Morning:** Push-up and sit-up routine (refer to Monday afternoon). **Afternoon:** Walk for 45–55 minutes.	Thurs
Morning: Run for 1.2 miles (2km). **Afternoon:** Push-up and sit-up routine (refer to Monday afternoon).	**Morning:** Walk for 45–55 minutes. **Afternoon:** Run for 1.4 miles (2.3km).	Fri
Morning: Walk for 40–50 minutes. **Afternoon:** Push-up and sit-up routine (refer to Monday afternoon).	Rest day.	Sat
Rest day.	**Morning:** Run for 1.4 miles (2.3km). **Afternoon:** Push-up and sit-up routine (refer to Monday afternoon).	Sun

DIET

Your fitness regime should include ensuring you eat a healthy diet. By eating healthily and cutting out excess carbohydrate, sugars, and salt, you will be better equipped to handle your fitness regime. You need to find the right balance between eating a sufficient amount to fuel your increased physical activity and creating enough of an energy deficit to prompt your body to burn any excess fat.

What to Avoid

You should consider reducing or cutting out altogether refined simple carbohydrates, such as sugar, contained in candies, desserts, baked goods, fruit juice, and sodas, and fats, contained in pastries, whole milk, butter, and food high in saturated fat. Rather than just cutting out items from your diet altogether, it can be helpful to think in terms of replacement. Here are some suggestions:

- Replace chocolate bars and other sugary snacks with fresh or dried fruit.

- Replace chips and salted nuts with salt-free alternatives or with fresh vegetables.
- Replace sugary drinks with carbonated water with a slice of fruit.
- Replace sugary breakfast cereals with lower sugar and salt varieties, or granola flavored with dried or fresh fruit such as dates or bananas.
- Think of alternatives to alcohol, such as mocktails, water or juice.
- Occasionally replace coffee and tea with low-caffeine or caffeine-free alternatives, such as green tea or chamomile.

US ARMY FITNESS GUIDE ADVICE ON NUTRITION

The US Armed Forces recognize how vital nutrition is to a successful fitness program and how important it is to get the right balance of foods into your diet. I have included this as a handy common-sense summary on diet and exercise.

US ARMY NUTRITION TIPS

— A meal should have the following proportions: two thirds vegetables, grains, or fruit, and one third low fat or lean protein from milk or meat.

— If you want to lose weight, cut down on calories while increasing exercise. Do this by having smaller portions and cutting down on foods with a high fat and sugar content.

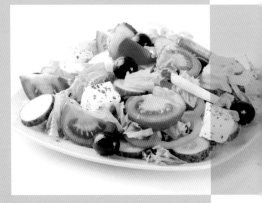

— To gain weight, increase calories while also increasing the amount of exercise. This means the weight you gain will be in the form of muscle, not fat.

— Take out of your diet fast, processed, and deep-fried foods, including sausages, burgers, fries, and pastries.

— Drink between eight and ten glasses of water per day.

— Although your food should provide all you need, take multivitamin and multimineral supplements (no more than 100% RDA) if necessary, to supplement nutritional requirements.

One of the keys to a good diet is awareness. This includes swapping unhealthy foods for healthy ones.

Fuel for the Machine

Just as you need to plan how much fuel to put in a car before a long journey, you need to plan your diet according to your energy expenditure. A healthy diet should involve cutting down on "empty" foods, or those that will give you a quick burst of energy followed by a rapid decline, and supplying your body with the right balance of nutrients to provide energy. Essential foods include:

- **Carbohydrates:** Bread, cereals, and pasta
- **Fats:** Milk, cheese, and butter
- **Protein:** Meat, fish, eggs, and nuts
- **Vitamins and minerals:** Found in vegetables, meat, and fruit

You also need fiber, which can be found in vegetables and grains. Fiber helps to keep your digestive system running efficiently and also helps to stave off hunger pangs by adding bulk to your diet.

Energy deficit

Rather than go on crash diets that inevitably run out of steam and only temporarily keep you off the bad food wagon, limit your calorie intake and force your body to burn excess fat in order to provide the energy it needs for the activity. This should be done in a planned way so that your body does not go into emergency mode and try to store up more fat to face starvation.

PLAN YOUR DIET ACCORDING TO YOUR ENERGY EXPENDITURE

A good way of gradually reducing excess fat is the long slow distance run (LSD, see page 30).

Pre-event meals

Although you may want to maintain a carbohydrate deficit (see above) as part of your weight-loss plan, you also need to have enough energy to complete your daily fitness regime. This means taking on enough complex carbohydrates for the job, so that you have sufficient glycogen in your liver to power the event. If you do not replenish glycogen, you run the risk of hypoglycemia (low blood sugar).

Morning training

You need to eat your main complex carbohydrate meal the night before to allow your body sufficient time to replenish glycogen stores. So eat a complex carbohydrate meal that includes pasta or something similar.

In the morning, start with a light breakfast, which may include:

- Granola with low-fat milk
- Fresh fruit or juice
- Muffin, bagel, toast, pancakes, or waffles
- Low-fat fruit yogurt

Afternoon training

Eat a complex carbohydrate meal the night before and in the morning before training. Then have a light lunch, which may include:

- Salad and low-fat dressing
- Turkey or chicken sandwiches
- Fruits
- Juice
- Low-fat crackers or rice cakes
- High carbohydrate nutritional bar

Evening training

Eat a complex carbohydrate breakfast and lunch, followed by a light meal that may include:

- Pasta with marinara sauce
- Rice with vegetables
- Light cheese pizza with vegetables
- Rice or noodle soup
- Baked potato
- Frozen yogurt

SAFETY

A military fitness program will be demanding on your body, especially at the beginning. It may be worth having a health check with your doctor to check any underlying heart problems, including arrhythmia or high blood pressure. Also check whether you have any underlying joint or back problems. If you have weight problems, you will need to give your body reasonable time to shed excess fat.

Resistance Training

Move your fitness regime forward gradually so that your body has time to make the underlying changes and take special care when doing resistance training such as weights. Overdoing weights can lead to heart strain as well as other injuries. When doing resistance exercise, you need to determine the appropriate combination of training volume and intensity, otherwise performance may be adversely affected and illness or injury may result. In a military fitness training program the body has to adapt to cardiovascular exercise as well as resistance training.

Get a Grip

If you are running on trails, which can be muddy, slippery, and uneven, it is worth investing in a pair of trail shoes. These have more rugged lugs than road shoes and will help you to stay upright when the going gets tough.

Hybrid shoes will work well on both the trail and the sidewalk. These are useful if you run on the sidewalk to get to the trail. Alternatively, have a pair of trail shoes and a pair of road shoes. The danger of using full trail shoes on a sidewalk, especially when it is wet, is that the lugs will slide on the surface.

Cold Weather Fitness Training

If it has been snowing and the snow is relatively soft, your trail shoes should be ideal. If the snow has frozen, it may be better to wear spikes, as even regular trail shoes may not break the surface.

- Wear enough layers of clothing to keep warm, taking into account the fact that your body temperature will rise and you will sweat while running. Wear a wicking layer close to the body so that sweat does not accumulate near your skin. When you stop and cool down, the sweat will freeze. It is a good idea to take a spare light fleece in a pack or tied round your waist.

- Wear a hat. You lose about 50 percent of body heat through your head.

- Wear sunglasses if necessary where there is sun reflected off snow, or to protect your eyes from snow flurries and cold air.

- Wear a mask or scarf over your face to prevent frostbite and also to warm the cold air before it hits your lungs. Freezing air can damage lungs, especially when inhaled in large quantities while running.

- Leave a map of your route with someone in case you have an injury.

BE SEEN, BE SAFE

If you are running or cycling in low-light conditions, make sure that you can be seen by wearing high-visibility clothing, or reflective armbands or vest. In winter, when it can get dark unexpectedly early, it is a good idea to take a small waist pack with some essentials and spares, such as:

☑ *Head torch*	☑ *Phone*	☑ *Gloves*
☑ *Waterproof jacket*	☑ *Whistle*	☑ *Water*
☑ *Light fleece*	☑ *Hat*	☑ *Cash*

Don't worry about the extra weight as it will contribute to your fitness!

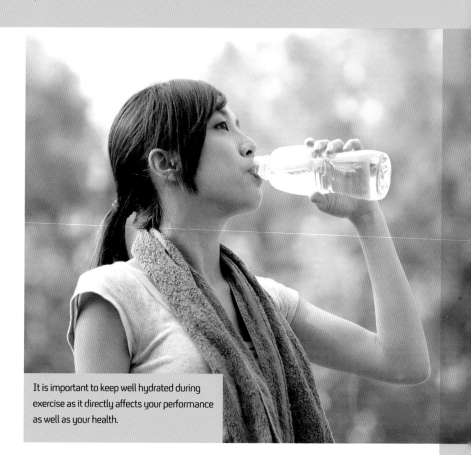

It is important to keep well hydrated during exercise as it directly affects your performance as well as your health.

Hot Weather Training

In hot weather, the danger is that you can overheat without being aware of it, become dehydrated by the joint effects of exercise and heat, and get sunstroke and sunburn.

- Wear light clothing, preferably with sun-resistant IV fabric
- Take a hat or cap
- Take sunglasses if necessary
- Wear sunscreen on exposed parts of your body
- Take plenty of water

US ARMY FITNESS GUIDE ADVICE ON INJURY PREVENTION

Depending on where you are exercising, the weather, and the level of fitness challenge, potential injuries always need to be taken into account. The US Army knows that prevention is the best cure.

Heat Injuries

If you experience any of the below symptoms of heat cramps, heat exhaustion, or heatstroke, stop your physical activity immediately.

Heat Cramps

— Muscular twitching
— Cramping
— Muscular spasms in arms, legs, or abdomen

Heat Exhaustion

— Excessive thirst
— Fatigue
— Lack of coordination
— Increased sweating
— Cool/wet skin
— Dizziness and/or confusion

Heatstroke

— No sweating
— Hot/dry skin
— Rapid pulse
— Rapid breathing
— Coma
— Seizure
— Dizziness and/or confusion
— Loss of consciousness

Cold Weather Injuries

When you get tired in cold climates and regions, your body's ability to produce heat is reduced and you may be in danger of getting hypothermia.

Hypothermia

— Shivering
— Loss of judgment
— Slurred speech
— Drowsiness
— Muscle weakness

Frostbite

— White or grayish-yellow skin patch
— Skin is firm or waxy
— Numb extremities, such as fingers, toes, and exposed skin

THE TESTS

In this part of the book you have the opportunity to test your fitness and see the results of all your hard work, focus, and determination. Remember, however, that even the baseline standards in military tests can be high. How you fare will depend in part on your age, stage of fitness, and the amount of time you have for training. So don't be put off if you don't make the grade! You can always try again.

These tests reflect the range of fitness expectations of a selection of military forces and units from around the world. The tests are organized on the basis of general entry requirements in the first section across army, navy, and air force. They start at general armed forces entry levels for various nations and move up to elite and special forces level, where the entry bar is placed higher. Real recruits usually have to pass the general entry before they can be considered for more advanced entry. So, see how you do in the first section and move on to the elite and special forces section once you have had a chance to hone your fitness! It goes without saying that military tests are closely monitored to obtain accurate results and to ensure health and safety standards are maintained. Some of the descriptions here are therefore for information purposes only: do not attempt anything that might be unsafe, especially where it comes to water-based tests.

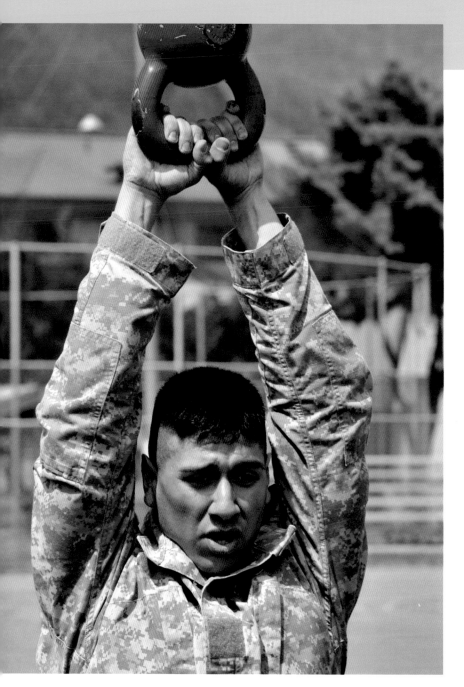

US ARMY

The US Army has no fitness test for recruits; it's only after being inducted that soldiers must pass the Army Physical Fitness Test (APFT), in order to graduate from Basic Training and enter Advanced Infantry Training. Soldiers are required to take the APFT twice a year for the rest of their active-duty career. (Reservists take it annually.) Failing two in a row can lead to dismissal from the Army, but soldiers are typically given remedial fitness training and allowed to retake the test.

Event	Assesses
Push-ups, 2 minutes	Arm, shoulder, and upper-body muscle strength and endurance
Sit-ups, 2 minutes	Abdominal and hip-flexor muscle strength and endurance
2-mile (3.2km) run, timed	Cardiovascular fitness

Scoring

The APFT has only three events, but an astonishingly complex set of scoring tables that adjust for age and gender. Performance in each event is scored on 100-point scale, so the maximum score is 300. The minimum scores needed to pass Basic Training are 50 on each event; once you're out of Basic, the minimums increase to 60 on each event. The Physical Fitness Badge is awarded to those who score 90 or greater on all three events.

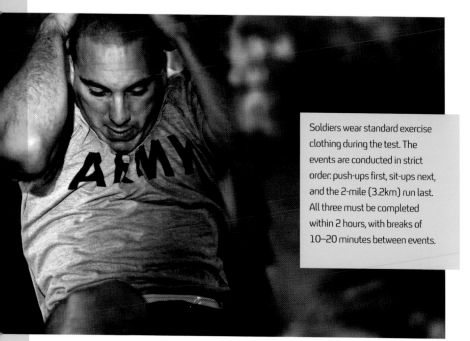

Soldiers wear standard exercise clothing during the test. The events are conducted in strict order: push-ups first, sit-ups next, and the 2-mile (3.2km) run last. All three must be completed within 2 hours, with breaks of 10–20 minutes between events.

Push-Ups

This is a timed drill to see how many push-ups you can perform in 2 minutes. An exercise mat may be used. The starting position is with the body and legs straight and the arms extended straight. Your head and neck may be held in any position you wish. The feet may be together or up to 12in (30cm) apart. The hands are placed on the ground at any comfortable distance. You may place your hands flat or use your fists. You may reposition your hands and feet during the test, but they must remain on the ground.

A successful push-up lowers your body until your upper arms are parallel to the ground, then raises your body back up so that your arms are straight. Your body and legs must remain rigid and straight from shoulders to ankles. You may touch your chest to the ground, but you may not bounce off it. You may rest during the test, but only in the "front leaning" or "altered front-leaning rest position," in which your back may be arched or sagging, and your knees may be slightly bent, but not to the extent that you take much weight off your arms.

Sit-Ups

This is another 2-minute drill in which you perform as many sit-ups as you can. An exercise mat may be used. The starting position is lying on your back, with your knees bent at a 90-degree angle and your feet flat on the ground. Your feet may be together or up to 12in (30cm) apart. Your hands must be clasped behind your head with the fingers interlocked. The backs of your hands must be on the ground. An assistant may hold your ankles. Raise your upper body to the vertical position or beyond. The base of your neck must be above or in front of the base of your spine. Your elbows may go inside or outside your knees and may, but need not, touch them.

To complete one sit-up, lower your body so that the bottom of your shoulder blades contact the ground. Your hands, arms, elbows, and head need not touch the ground. Your knees may not exceed a 90-degree angle and your heels must remain in contact with the ground. Your hands must remain in contact with the back of your head. Your fingers must remain interlocked.

You may wiggle your body to help attain the vertical position. You may not: bow or arch your back, bounce off the ground; raise your buttocks or heels off the ground; push with any part of your arms or hands against the ground; swing your arms to create momentum. You may rest only in the "up" position, but you may not use your arms to brace or lock yourself against your legs. As long as you attempt to raise yourself from the down position, the event will continue.

Most failures of form result in only that attempt not being counted. However, resting in a non-approved posture or swinging your arms for momentum will terminate the event.

2-Mile (3.2km) Run

This event is a timed 2-mile (3.2km) run, with participants striving to achieve the shortest possible time. The course may be a running track or any other measured course with good footing, minimal slope, and a clear unobstructed path. Walking is permitted. You may be paced by another runner, but of course you can not be helped by being pushed, pulled, or supported. Bystanders are permitted to cheer and to call out elapsed times.

RANGER FITNESS TEST

Rangers are a special forces unit of the US Army, although members of other military branches and even some from other countries attend Ranger School for training. Women will be allowed to train at Ranger School for the first time in 2015, meeting the same physical requirements as male soldiers.

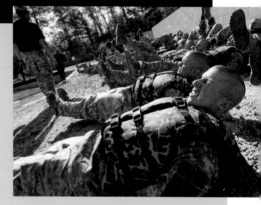

Ranger training is beyond rigorous—it is extreme—involving lengthy, realistic survival and battle scenarios on short rations and little sleep in desert, swamp and mountain environments. So demanding is the regime that less than half of the students pass, and those who do are often so physically taxed that it takes months to fully recover.

Compared to the full course, the Ranger Physical Fitness Test is a cakewalk, but it's still a difficult challenge even to most soldiers. It's pass/fail, with the following minimum requirements:

— **Push-ups:** 49 in 2 minutes, as per the Army Physical Fitness Test.
— **Sit-ups:** 59 in 2 minutes, as per the Army Physical Fitness Test.

— **Chin-ups:** 6 required. Chin-Ups are of the "dead hang" sort, requiring that the arms be fully extended between every rep. The grip is overhand, with the palms facing forward and thumbs around the bar. The chin must be raised above the bar. The legs must remain straight and no lower body movement is permitted. There is no time restriction.

— **5-mile (8km) run:** 40 minutes. The course is cross-country on gentle, rolling terrain.

BRITISH ARMY

The British Army is a highly trained national force that protects British territory but is also deployed on a wide range of simultaneous missions in different parts of the world. The British Army can deploy battalions on a large scale or provide elite and special forces for more focused missions. It is also involved in humanitarian work, including peace support operations and training.

Once recruits have completed their medical at the Army Development and Selection Centre (ADSC), they are asked to carry out two days of fitness testing. The tests for British Army entry vary according to which branch of the army the recruit plans to serve in. The standards are higher for infantry than for other roles and they are especially high for elite regiments such as the Paratroop Regiment.

The Real Deal

The British Army have added a flavor of realism to their entrance fitness test. A range of strength and stamina tests have to be undertaken, which include carrying weights such as a jerrican: the sort of thing you would expect to do in a real-life military scenario.

The static or power bag lift

This is a practical test to see if you can lift weights. For example, you may need to lift a heavy backpack into the back of a truck. Power bag weights start at 33lb (15kg) and move up to 88lb (40kg). The weighted bag of 33lb has to be lifted to a height of 4¾ft (1.45m).

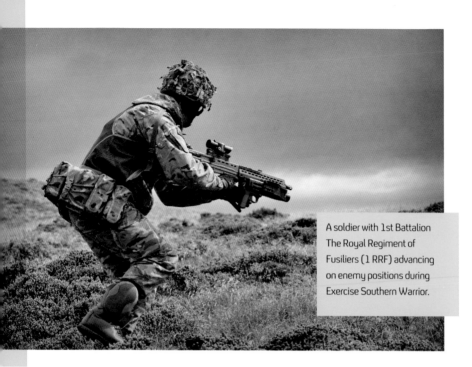

A soldier with 1st Battalion The Royal Regiment of Fusiliers (1 RRF) advancing on enemy positions during Exercise Southern Warrior.

Jerrican test

Again, this reflects the sort of practical activity a recruit may be involved in on any day in their military life. The recruit carries two 45lb (20kg) water containers over a course of 130yd (120m) without stopping. The course has to be completed in 2 minutes or less. This tests the recruit's whole body strength and determination.

Push-ups

A minimum of 44 in 2 minutes.

Sit-ups

A minimum of 50 in 2 minutes.

1.5-mile (2.4km) run

The aim of the run is to achieve your best time but the absolute maximim is 09:30 minutes. The run is on a level ground with a stable running surface.

CANADIAN ARMED FORCES

A test takes place during the first week of basic training to assess each candidate's level of physical fitness. The candidate must pass the test to continue with basic training. The tests are designed to reflect typical military activity on operations. The sprint with a drop-down every 33ft (10m) mirrors the sort of maneuvers soldiers would have to undertake when under fire. The sandbag drag and carry again reflects the military reality of building a shell scrape or trench for protection.

The test has three main parts:

- An 88yd (80m) sprint, dropping to a prone position every 11yd (10m). This exercise can be easily practiced and is an excellent test of overall fitness and quick recovery, as it is very testing to get down on your front in the middle of a run.

- A 22yd (20m) sandbag drag, during which you must carry one 44lb (20kg) sandbag and pull a minimum of four sandbags on the floor. This test will help your body to adjust to irregular strains while running.

It strengthens your legs as you pull on the extra weight, and also trains your torso and arms to manage shifting weight.

- A 22yd (20m) shuttle run to measure aerobic fitness. The shuttle run is a recurrent theme in this book. The fact that it keeps coming up testifies to its effectiveness as a fitness test.

The table on the page opposite outlines what will be expected of you when tested.

Test performance objectives

Test	Performance Objective
1. 88yd (80m) sprint	51 sec
2. Sandbag drag	Complete without stopping
3. 22yd (20m) shuttle run (bleep test)	Men under 35: 6.0 Men over 35: 5.0 Women under 35: 4.0 Women over 35: 3.0

If recruits fail to pass the whole set but meet one or more of the three items, they might be eligible for further training at the Warrior Preparation Company at the Canadian Forces Leadership and Recruit School. They are then given a maximum of 90 days to pass all parts of the test.

Basic Training

The tests outlined above are designed to prepare the recruit for basic training, which involves some of the following elements. The average day starts at 5:00 a.m. and ends at 11:00 p.m and includes physical training, marching, classes, and practical sessions on a variety of military subjects.

Obstacle course

The obstacle course includes scaling 6.5 and 13ft (2 and 4m) walls, climbing a 13ft (4m) netting apparatus, and crossing a 13ft (4m) ditch while hanging from a set of monkey bars. These activities require good upper-body strength.

Swimming

The military swim test involves jumping into a pool wearing a life jacket and swimming 55yd (50m). Other training includes somersaulting into the water without a life jacket, treading water for 2 minutes, and then swimming 22yd (20m).

Physical training

Field exercises include 8-mile (13km) marches in full combat gear and meeting the forces' minimum physical fitness standard, which is a requirement for passing basic training. Physical training at basic training includes:

- Skill and strength development
- Running progressively longer distances up to 3.7 miles (6km)
- Completing marches of various lengths in full combat gear

BELGIAN ARMED FORCES

Belgium has three armed services: navy, army, and air force, along with elite forces of commandos and special forces. Belgian forces are highly trained and they demand very high standards of their recruits. The Belgian Armed Forces carry out standard physical assessment tests for all ranks and there are supplementary tests for those who wish to enter the Ecole Royale Militaire (ERM), or Royal Military Academy.

The Standard Tests

You must obtain a 50 percent mark for the anaerobic tests and 50 percent for the aerobic tests. The percentages are worked out from a fairly complex scoring system.

Anaerobic capacity

Test 1: Push-ups *(pompage)*

- Support yourself with your hands and rest your legs on your toes (males) or knees (females)
- Hold your body in a straight line
- Turn your hands slightly inward
- Bend your arms at 90 degrees to lower yourself toward the ground
- The test lasts 1 minute

Test 2: Sit-ups *(abdominaux)*

- Lie on your back
- Bend your knees at 90 degrees
- Your feet should be held down
- Your fingers should be touching your ears
- Using your abdominal muscles, lift yourself up until your elbows touch your upper thighs
- The test lasts 1 minute

Aerobic capacity

A 1.5-mile (2,4km) run. The minimum time for men (age 20–29) is 11:40 minutes. For women of the same age it is 14:25 minutes.

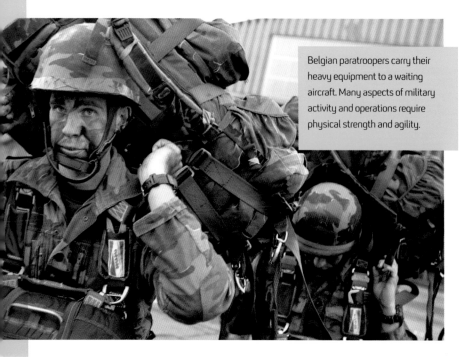

Belgian paratroopers carry their heavy equipment to a waiting aircraft. Many aspects of military activity and operations require physical strength and agility.

Ecole Royale Militaire (ERM)

The Belgian Royal Military Academy provides university-level education for officers in the Belgian navy, army, air force, and medical services. The additional tests for those entering the Ecole Royale Militaire (ERM) are:

- A 6.2-mile (10km) run
- A 437yd (400m) swim
- Pull-ups (20)
- Rope climbs (10)
- Sit-ups (20)

You must obtain a score of 50 percent across the additional tests. Once you have passed into the academy the tests become gradually more demanding.

DANISH ARMED FORCES

The Danish physical fitness test is the result of a thorough review of training requirements, based largely on the experiences and requirements of Danish soldiers serving in Afghanistan. Having reviewed the physical demands from the ground upward, they produced the Danish Concept of Military Physical Training. The new concept is designed to promote fitness and overall good health while also minimizing the risk of injuries.

Danish Military Physical Training

The basis of the concept is that a soldier needs good all-round physical capability in order to cope with the wide variety of challenges they face, including patrolling, equipment, climate, changes in the availability of adequate food and nutrition, variations in terrain, and challenges posed by contact with the enemy. The aim is to create military athletes who are equal to the physical, psychological, and tactical challenges that they face.

The Danish Military Physical Training concept focuses on core muscular strength as well as aerobic and anaerobic capacity. By increasing physical performance, energy levels are also increased, while fatigue and the risk of injuries are reduced.

Circuit training is considered an excellent way to build up the body's adaptability and robustness, making it easier to adapt to a variety of demands.

Developing the full range of military physical fitness takes time. The following are broad estimates for the time it takes to develop:

- Aerobic and anaerobic capacity: one to two months
- Muscular strength: two months
- Bone structure: five months
- Ligaments, joints, and connective tissue: seven months

Training, therefore, has to take into account the time it takes for these adaptations to take place. The Danish Armed Forces grade their physical fitness tests according to the demands of the role. The highest grade is for special forces and commandos and the next for infantry soldiers, engineers, combat medics, and similar roles.

The Danish Military Physical Training concept is divided into two broad categories:
1. **Core Test:** This is used to assess overall core fitness in the army, navy, and air force. The recommended level of fitness is 3.
2. **The Danish Armed Forces Physical Test:** This is divided into blocks A, B, C, and D for the army and A, B, and C for both the navy and air force.

Soldiers are graded on a scale between zero and 5. Apart from formal tests, unit commanders are also able to test soldiers at any time.

The Core Test

1. Back
- Lie over a box with your hip two finger widths over the edge
- Your legs must be held by a companion
- Hold your body straight with your back muscles
- Take your arms off the ground
- Maintain a straight horizontal position for as long as possible or a maximum of 165 seconds

2. Ninety percent static sit-up
- Lie on your back and bring your feet back so that your legs and hips are at a 90-degree angle
- Your feet should be held down by a partner
- Raise your torso upward with your hands folded over your chest

3–4. Sidebridge left/right
- Place your elbow and forearm on the floor
- Ensure your elbow is directly below your armpit
- Place your feet on top of each other, stacked in parallel
- Raise your body to the test position
- Hold the position for a maximum of 120 seconds

5–6. Backbridge left/right

- Lie on your back with both feet on the ground
- Fold your arms over your chest
- Push one leg out straight
- Raise yourself on your other leg
- Push your hip upward

Try this position on both left and right for a maximum of 90 seconds.

7. Lunges

- Stand straight holding a 44lb (20kg) weight across your shoulders
- Step forward with one leg, resting your back foot on your toes
- Move your hips downward until the rear knee is at least 4in (10cm) from the ground
- Keep your back straight and your knees stable

Repeat the test for as long as you can on alternating legs, or for a maximum of 60 times. You should not attempt any tests without formal training or guidance, especially the more challenging ones, as this could lead to injury.

Aerobic Fitness Tests

Block A is designed to test how well your body absorbs, transports, and consumes oxygen while you perform aerobic distance running. You can choose one of the following two tests:

1. 12-minute run

You will be tested on how far you can run in 12 minutes. The test should be conducted outdoors on a 437yd (400m) running course. It helps to mark the test course at every 55 or 110yd (50 or 100m).

2. Yo-Yo UH 1

A 66ft (20m) shuttle-run/bleep test. This test is held in a gymnasium between two marked lines which are 66ft (20m) apart. You need to touch the lines with your feet when you hear the beep. As the intervals between the beeps get progressively shorter, you have to run faster to reach the line before the next beep. The test score is the level you last started before you were unable to keep up with the recording.

Danish Military Physical Tests

Level	1. Back	2. Static sit-up	3. Sidebridge left	4. Sidebridge right	5. Backbridge left	6. Backbridge right	7. Lunges with 45lb (20kg)
5	155 sec	135 sec	120 sec	120 sec	90 sec	90 sec	60 reps
4	150 sec	120 sec	105 sec	105 sec	75 sec	75 sec	50 reps
3	135 sec	105 sec	90 sec	90 sec	60 sec	60 sec	40 reps
2	120 sec	90 sec	75 sec	75 sec	45 sec	45 sec	40 reps
1	105 sec	75 sec	60 sec	60 sec	30 sec	30 sec	20 reps

Aerobic and Anaerobic Fitness Tests

In Block B you will be assessed in aerobic and anaerobic distance, i.e., your body's ability to tolerate fatigue and repeatedly perform high-intensity tasks. You can choose one of the following two tests:

Yo-Yo IR 1

This test is similar to Yo-Yo UH 1, but it includes 10-second pauses between each running interval. As the intervals between the start and finish beeps become progressively shorter, you will have to run faster each time to reach the line before the beep. The test score is the level you last started before you were unable to keep up with the recording.

The Danish Military Speed Test

The Danish Military Speed Test was invented by the Center for Physical Training. You can take this simple test anywhere and at any time.

Mark two lines 66ft (20m) apart. The test consists of running between the two lines as many times as possible in 30 seconds, followed by 30 seconds of rest. Repeat the cycle 10 times. Then add up the number of completed rounds and the result is your test score.

Muscular Fitness Tests

Block C rates your muscular strength, namely your body's ability to repeatedly generate a large amount of strength over a short period of time. There are five tests designed to assess your overall muscular fitness level. The tests are designed to reflect the physical challenges of soldiers patrolling with heavy weights such as backpacks and other equipment.

Lunges

- Stand straight holding a weight of between 22 and 110lb (10 and 50kg) across your shoulders
- Step forward with one leg
- Rest your back foot on the toes
- Move your hips downward until your rear knee is at least 4in (10cm) from the ground
- Keep your back straight and your knees stable

Repeat the test for as long as you can on alternating legs or for a maximum of 60 times.

Dips

- Grasp the horizontal bars of an appropriate piece of gym equipment
- Lower the upper body until your upper arms are at 90 degrees to the ground

> # THE TESTS ARE DESIGNED TO REFLECT THE PHYSICAL CHALLENGES FACED BY SOLDIERS

- Return to the start position
- Repeat one to eight times

You can use a weight of 22lb (10kg), depending on the test score.

Pull-ups

- Grasp the bar with an overhand grip
- Bend your legs slightly
- Keep your body and legs stable
- Pull up until chin passes over the beam
- Lower body to start position

Repeat the test between one and eight times. Optional weight of 22lb (10kg).

Deadlifts

- Place your hands on the barbell bar
- Place your feet shoulder-width apart
- Keeping your arms straight, perform a leg press until the body is straight
- Lower your body to the start position

The weight must touch the floor prior to each lift, although you cannot rest the weight on the floor between the lifts. Repeat six to eight times with no weight or with a weight of between 88 and 220lb (40 and 100kg).

The plank

*This part should only be carried out with a qualified assistant due to risk of injury.

- Get down on the ground
- Keep your forearms shoulder-width apart
- Raise your body in the "plank" position, supporting your body on your forearms and toes
- *A 0–45lb (0–20kg) weight should be placed over the lower back
- Maintain the position for 60–120 seconds

Functional Tests

Block D is designed to measure your aerobic and functional motor skills.

The tests include:

- A 1.2-mile (2km) march (no running)
- A 547yd (500m) military obstacle course
- Another 1.2-mile (2km) march

You should carry equipment weighing 55lb (25kg) (not including uniform and boots).

Obstacle Course

Recruits must tackle the following obstacles on the course. (If you want to try similar obstacles, it would be advisable for health and safety reasons to find a civilian obstacle course that you can attempt under supervision.)

- Rope ladder
- Sloping wall with rope
- Irish table
- Four steps of beam
- Pit
- Vertical ladder

FINNISH ARMED FORCES

The Finnish Armed Forces advise that all potential recruits begin a suitable fitness program without delay. The Finns say that if you are able to run over 1.8 miles (2.9km) in 12 minutes, you are in excellent physical shape. If you run 1.8 miles in more than 12 minutes, you should start a comprehensive exercise program as soon as possible.

Training

The Finns rightly point out that military training includes a great deal of walking. They point out that stamina and muscle strength are the two basic components of military training. Apart from increasing walking in general, they also recommend Nordic walking, running, swimming, cycling, rowing, roller-skating, and cross-country skiing. They recommend that stamina exercises are done one or two times per week. They also recommend ball sports and other team sports to develop coordination and teamwork. In some form or other, military training always involves teamwork; being able to anticipate and read the mind of your teammates is an important skill.

The importance of warm-ups and cool-downs is also highlighted, along with easy exercising that helps the muscles to readjust after a hard session. This may include walking, gentle jogging, or cycling at an easy pace. They also recommend massage and a good diet, along with plenty of water.

When assessing military fitness requirements, the Finnish Defence Forces (FDF) took account of the reduction

Finnish Defense Forces' 12-minute fitness classification

Classification	Male	Female
Weak	Less than 2,133yd (1,950m)	Less than 1,860yd (1,700m)
Poor	2,133–2,734yd (1,950–2,500m)	1,860–2,406yd (1,700–2,200m)
Satisfactory	2,734–2,953yd (2,500–2,700m)	2,406–2,625yd (2,200–2,400m)
Good	2,953–3,171yd (2,700–2,900m)	2,625–2,843yd (2,400–2,600m)
Commendable	3,171–3,390yd (2,900–3,100m)	2,843–3,062yd (2,600–2,800m)
Excellent	More than 3,390yd (3,100m)	More than 3,062yd (2,800m)

in fitness of potential candidates in comparison with previous years. This means that there is more work to be done in bringing young men and women up to the required fitness standard.

Despite the advances in technological warfare, the physical demands remain the same. Military environments often include a variety of stressors, including prolonged physical exertion, unpredictable food and water supplies, and extreme temperatures. Another point is that during operations physical performance can deteriorate and there is little time for either maintaining or improving physical performance. This underlines the importance of developing excellent fitness before operations. The Finnish are aware that physical fitness also promotes good health, making it more likely that soldiers will endure periods of difficulty and deprivation. There is a recognition of endurance training as well as strength training. To improve aerobic fitness and muscle strength, periodization should be used to avoid interference in strength development caused by concurrent endurance and strength training.

Fitness testing in the FDF is compulsory on an annual basis for all professional soldiers. The FDF monitor the physical fitness of their staff, including aerobic capacity and muscle fitness tests, as well as body height, weight, and waist circumference.

Professional soldiers also need to pass field duty fitness tests, including shooting, marching, and orienteering tests. Before physical fitness testing begins, all candidates receive a health screening.

Aerobic Fitness Test

12-minute run

You should perform the 12-minute run outside, although it can be performed indoors on a treadmill if necessary. You should gradually increase your speed throughout the run, which is a test of your best effort.

A reasonable goal is 2 miles (3.2km) in 12 minutes, which means running 1 mile (1.6km) in 6 minutes. You can break it down further to make it easier for yourself: ½ mile (0.8km) in 3 minutes and ¼ of a mile (0.4km) in 90 seconds. Psychologically, it helps to be aware of these sub-goals so that you don't run too fast at the beginning and tire yourself out too quickly. As you achieve your sub-goals, you will realize that you are on the right track.

Bicycle ergometer test

The standard test is to pedal on a cycle ergometer at a constant workload for 7 minutes. The initial workload of the test is 50 watts, increased by 25 watts every second minute until exhaustion. Heart rate is continuously recorded using a heart rate monitor. VO_2 peak is normally measured at the point where you become exhausted. In general, the lower your heart rate, the more fit you are.

UKK walk test

This test is used to establish your baseline fitness without putting yourself under too much pressure. Walk as fast as possible for 1.2 miles (2km) in a flat area. The result of your performance should be recorded as VO_2 max calculated on the basis of your age, gender, height, weight, and the time taken to cover the distance. Your heart rate is measured at the end of the walk. The formula is quite complex so it would need to be carried out in a controlled environment with professional help or on a suitable running machine.

Muscle Fitness Tests

These include sit-ups, push-ups, and the standing long jump. The sit-up test is used to measure the endurance of the abdominal muscles and hip flexors. The push-up test is used to measure the physical performance of the upper-body muscles. The standing long jump is used to measure the explosive force of the leg extensor muscles.

Sit-ups

- Lie on your back with your hands behind your neck, elbows pointing forward
- Flex your knees at 90 degrees
- Your ankles should be held
- Lift your upper body and touch your knees with your elbows

The test result will be the number of sit-ups that you can complete in 60 seconds.

Push-ups

- Get down on the floor with fully extended arms and a straight torso
- Place your hands shoulder-width apart, fingers pointing forward
- Place your legs in a parallel push-up position
- Lower your body until your elbows are at an angle of 90 degrees

The result of this test is the number of push-ups completed in 60 seconds.

Standing long jump

- Stand with legs together
- Use arms and upper body to create a powerful explosive forward momentum

Repeat three times. The result of the test is the best jump measured in meters.

Fitness Tests for Field Dut

In order to estimate soldiers' fitness for field duty annually, basic field tests including marching, orienteering, and shooting are used by the FDF. The fitness for field duty index is based on these tests. In addition, almost all branches of the armed forces have their own specific task-related field fitness tests, which are not described here.

Marching

This test is used to evaluate your ability to maintain your performance both during and after prolonged physical strain. The test is carried out in cross-country terrain and involves completing either a 15.5-mile (25km) walk, 18.6 miles (30km) of cross-country skiing, or 50 miles (80km) of cycling while carrying combat gear and a rifle. The test must be completed in 6 hours.

Other elements include orienteering (a run of at least 3.1 miles/5km in tough forest and cross-country terrain or ski orienteering in the winter), shooting tests, and swimming, including a life-saving swim. If you are interested in trying outdoor activities such as orienteering, contact a local club.

FRENCH ARMED FORCES

The French Armed Forces are arguably the most successful in the world in terms of battles won. They have a wide range of units across the navy, army, air force, and Gendarmerie Nationale. The general standard entry test for the French Armed Forces has its own unique qualities and, like many things French, is different to many other standard entry tests. The standard French Armed Forces physical entry tests are run by the Département Evaluation Information (DEI).

The French have created a form of mini obstacle course in order to provide the testers with an overview of how the candidate performs under timed pressure. Although conventional tests such as pull-ups and sit-ups are included in the test, the emphasis is very much on overall coordination alongside physical fitness. The logic here is that one of the measures of fitness is recovery. If you are fit, you should be able to stay focused when asked to perform exercises such as ball throwing at a target in the midst of other physical activity.

Test sportif de Luc Léger

This is the bleep test. Male candidates must achieve level 8 and females level 7.

Obstacle Course

An agility, strength, and coordination course consisting of the following:

- **Plinth (gym horse):** You must jump over it with hands on the top, passing both legs over the top.

- **Long jump:** Jump before the front edge of the mat and land with one foot over a marked line on the mat.

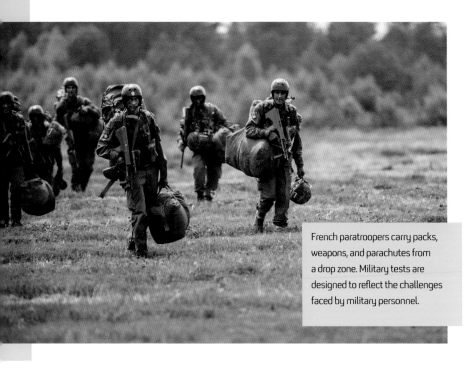

French paratroopers carry packs, weapons, and parachutes from a drop zone. Military tests are designed to reflect the challenges faced by military personnel.

- **Sit-ups:** These are done from the upright position in a gym structure, allowing you to pull your knees up to your chest (15 times for men and 10 times for women).

- **Bar:** Walk across a bar, maintaining balance.

- **Rings:** You must hop into different color rings with one leg (left leg in red rings; right leg in yellow rings). Your feet must land in the center of the rings and not touch the edges.

- **Ball throwing:** Onto a target 30 feet (9m) away.

- **Pull-ups:** Holding your chin above the bar for as long as possible. Male candidates should do a minimum of four pull-ups and women one pull-up.

Maximum points are gained if you complete the course in under 2:15 minutes.

IRISH DEFENSE FORCES

The Irish Defense Force consist of a navy, army, and air corps. Apart from national security, the IDF are often involved in peacekeeping, peace support, and humanitarian relief operations around the world. To join the Irish Defense Forces you need to pass a physical fitness test and thereafter undergo an annual physical fitness test.

Defense Forces' Induction Fitness Test

The Physical Fitness test is designed to assess the candidate's current level of physical fitness and their capacity to undergo military training. It is composed of three aspects.

Body composition

Assessment of percentage of body fat, using the body mass index (BMI) test and skinfold caliper test (if necessary). Calipers are usually applied to a pinched area of body skin to measure the amount of fat. The measurement is based on a calculation of the width of skin pinched in millimeters and fat density, which is then converted into a percentage. For athletic males, a score of 60–80 percent is good; for women 70–85 percent is good. Individuals who score in excess of 2¾-in/70mm (males) or 3⅛in/80mm (females) on the skinfold caliper test will not be permitted to take the test.

General information on BMI

Body Mass Index checks whether the relationship between height and weight is a healthy one. For example: If a male recruit is 5'11" (1.80m) and weighs 188lb (85kg), his BMI is about 26. If a female recruit is 5'4" (1.63m) and weighs 132lb (60kg), her BMI is about 23.

Please note the following in relation to the BMI readings:

- **BMI of <20:** May be associated with health problems for some people. It may be a good idea to consult your doctor for advice.
- **BMI of 20–25:** Good health for most people. This is the range you want to stay in.
- **BMI of 25–29.9:** Indicates overweight and may be associated with health problems for some people.

Local Muscular Endurance

Each candidate undergoes a local muscular endurance test where they are required to complete 20 push-ups and 20 sit-ups, each within a minute.

Push-ups

- Place your hands slightly more than shoulder-width apart
- Hands must remain in the original position
- Your body must be held in a straight line from the shoulders to hips to heels
- Your feet may be up to 12in (30cm) apart
- Don't twist your body or lock out your elbows

NB: Females may do modified push-ups.

Modified push-ups

- These are push-ups done from the knees
- Hands must remain in the original position
- Your body must be held in a straight line from the shoulders to hips to heels
- Do not drop your head, twist your body, or lock out your elbows

Aerobic Capacity

Each candidate is required to complete an aerobic capacity test which involves running a certain distance in a given time. The table below outlines the times for males and females.

Aerobic capacity requirements (1.5 miles/2.4km)

	Max time allowed
Male	11:40 min
Female	13:10 min

LUXEMBOURG ARMED FORCES

As a landlocked country, Luxembourg has no navy. It also does not have an official air force, though it does possess military aircraft. The main military force is therefore the army, which is part of the NATO force. The Luxembourg Army is also incorporated into the Beluga Force, which is a joint force under Belgian command.

To join the Luxembourg Armed Forces recruits are required to pass a variety of physical, psychological, and medical tests. The design of the tests is in line with the growing emphasis on practical exercises that test overall coordination and movement. The sprint test, for example, not only measures raw sprinting speed but also overall body fitness as the candidate must raise themselves from a prone position on the ground before the sprint.

The tests include:

- **Throwing a 6.6lb (3kg) ball:** From a sitting position, throw the ball as far as you can. You get three attempts.
- **Sit-ups:** Lie on your back with your legs bent and your hands behind your head. Complete as many sit-ups as possible in 2 minutes, touching your head against your knees and lying back down again.
- **Long jump:** Bend your knees and jump with both feet as far as you can. You get three attempts and the longest jump will be counted.

Success criteria for the aptitude test

Points	Throwing a 6.6lb (3kg) ball		Sit-ups (in 2 min)		Long jump		Sprint test 26yd (24 m)		Push-ups (in 2 min)		1.5-mile (2.4km) run	
	M	F	M	F	M	F	M	F	M	F	M	F
20	≥ 7.8yd (7.1m)	≥ 6.8yd (6.2m)	≥ 74	≥ 68	≥ 2.7yd (2.5m)	≥ 2.6yd (2.4m)	≤ 4.2 sec	≤ 4.4 sec	≥ 64	≥ 39	≤ 9:45 min	≤ 12:15 min
10	≥ 5.7yd (5.2m)	≥ 5.4yd (4.9m)	≥ 45	≥ 39	≥ 2.7yd (2.5m)	≥ 2.1yd (1.9m)	≤ 5.2 sec	≤ 5.4 sec	≥ 36	≥ 24	≤ 12:15 min	≤ 14:30 min
1	≥ 3.8yd (3.5m)	≥ 3.1yd (2.8m)	≥ 20	≥ 18	≥ 1.7yd (1.55m)	≥ 1.6yd (1.45m)	≤ 5.8 sec	≤ 6.0 sec	≥ 18	≥ 10	≤ 14:30 min	≤ 15:50 min

- **Push-ups:** Your straight body should be supported by your toes and your hands. Complete as many push-ups as possible in 2 minutes.
- **1.5-mile (2.4km) run:** Complete the distance as fast as you can on an athletic track.

Sprint

Lie flat on the ground on your back with your head nearest to the start line. On the signal to start, get up off the ground and sprint as fast as you can to the finish point. A second person with a stopwatch should time you.

To successfully complete the military physical fitness test recruits must complete all six tests and gain at least 10 points in the sit-ups and push-ups and at least one point in all the other tests. An average of 10 out of 20 points must be obtained overall.

THE SPRINT TEST NOT ONLY MEASURES RAW SPRINTING SPEED BUT ALSO OVERALL BODY FITNESS

NEW ZEALAND DEFENSE FORCE

The New Zealand Defense Force (NZDF) is made up of a navy, army, and air force; it has about 14,000 personnel. There are about 9,000 regular service personnel, 2,200 in the reserve forces, and the remainder are civil personnel. The New Zealand Defense Force protects New Zealand from external threats, protects its economic zone, provides support for its ally Australia, and is also involved in peace support and humanitarian operations worldwide.

NZ Army Fitness Test

The Entry Fitness Level (EFL) test must be completed by recruits on induction day. The requirements for the test are given in the table below.

Defense Forces' 12-minute fitness classification

	Run 1.5 miles (2.4km)	Curl-ups	Push-ups
Male	12 min	45	15
Female	14 min	35	8

New Zealand Navy

To enter the Royal New Zealand Navy a recruit will need to complete a multi-stage fitness test (bleep test, see page 166) as well as push-ups. Once a recruit has passed through to basic training, they have to pass a swimming test. This involves a 55yd (50m) swim in overalls and gym shoes as well as treading water for 3 minutes. Ongoing fitness training once recruits have passed into the navy include:

- Carrying a 45lb (20kg) weight for four 16yd (15m) shuffles in less than 45 seconds
- Dragging a dummy body 16yd (15m) in less than 30 seconds

Six-Week Fitness Challenge

Like many armed forces, the NZDF recommends that potential recruits start preparing as soon as possible for entrance fitness tests. Their Six-Week Fitness Challenge has been devised for those who either do not exercise at all or who do very little exercise.

Six-week fitness challenge

	Week 1	Week 2	Week 3	Week 4	Week5	Week 6
Run	Mon, Weds, Fri: Run at a comfortable pace for 20 min. Jog/walk as an alternative.	Mon, Weds, Fri: Run at a comfortable pace for 25 min. Jog/walk as an alternative.	Mon, Fri: Run at a comfortable pace for 25 min. Weds: Run 1.5 miles (2.4km) in 12:30 min.	Mon, Thur: Run at a comfortable pace for 30 minutes. Tue, Fri: Run 1.5 miles (2.4km) in 12 min.	Tue, Fri: Run at a comfortable pace for 30 minutes. Mon, Thur: Run 1.5 miles (2.4km) in 11:30 minutes.	Tue: Run at a comfortable pace for 30 min. Mon, Fri: Run 1.5 miles (2.4km) in 11 min. Sat: Run at a comfortable pace for 20 min.
Push-ups	Tue, Thur, Sat: 5–10 × 3 sets	Tue, Thur, Sat: 8–12 × 3 sets	Tue, Thur: 10–15 × 3 sets	Tue, Thur, Sat: 15–20 × 3 sets	Tue, Thur, Sat: 20 × 3 sets	Mon, Wed, Fri: 25+ × 1 sets
Curl-ups	Tue, Thur, Sat: 10–15 × 3 sets	Tue, Thur, Sat: 10–15 × 3 sets	Tue, Thur: 15 × 3 sets	Tue, Thur, Sat: 15–20 × 3 sets	Tue, Thur, Sat: 20 × 3 sets	Mon, Wed, Fri: 20 × 2 sets
Half squats	Tue, Thur, Sat: 10–15 × 3 sets	Tue, Thur, Sat: 12–15 × 3 sets	Tue, Thur: 15–20 × 3 sets	Tue, Thur, Sat: 15–20 × 3 sets	Tue, Thur, Sat: 20 × 3 sets	Mon, Wed, Fri: 20 × 2 sets
Back arches	Tue, Thur, Sat: 10–15 × 3 sets	Tue, Thur, Sat: 12–15 × 3 sets	Tue, Thur: 15 × 3 sets	Tue, Thur, Sat: 15 × 3 sets	Tue, Thur, Sat: 15 × 3 sets	Mon, Wed, Fri: 15 × 3 sets
Pull-ups	N/a	N/a	N/a	Attempt	Tue, Thur, Sat: Attempt	Mon, Wed, Fri: Attempt

The 100 Club

The New Zealand Army have a "100 Club" for serving officers and soldiers. Membership involves meeting the following fitness standards:

	Run 1.5 miles (2.4km)	Curl-ups	Push-ups
Male	8 min	130	55
Female	10:05 min	118	36

Royal New Zealand Air Force

In the Royal New Zealand Air Force, recruits are required to complete a 3.1-mile (5km) march carrying 45lb (20kg) in 42 minutes (male) or 44:30 minutes (female) in the 16–29 age bracket.

NORWEGIAN ARMED FORCES

Aerobic fitness is important for your ability to endure physical and psychological stress. Great emphasis is placed on this in the Norwegian Armed Forces fitness testing program. The physical fitness tests are designed for new candidates for military training but there are also tests for already enlisted personnel, including a treadmill running test and isometric tests to measure arm and leg strength.

Military Personnel

The tests consist of a 1.9-mile (3km) run to assess aerobic fitness, and pull-ups, sit-ups, and push-ups to assess muscle fitness. The tests are performed three times within three weeks of entering. The required test scores are 2 for the 1.9-mile (3km) run and an average of 2 for the three muscle-fitness tests.

1.9-mile (3km) run

This run must be done on a track, road, or trail. The test circuit should be mostly flat, with a maximum rise of 33ft (10m). The course should be marked with signs at intervals of 547yd (500m).

Pull-ups

Men

- Hang vertically from a gymnastics beam
- Place your hands in an overhand grip
- Take your feet off the floor
- Raise your body until your chin is above the upper part of the beam
- Lower yourself until your arms are fully extended

Keep going for as long as you can with calm, controlled movements. If you cannot do a full pull-up, don't worry as your muscles will have got the message from your efforts and you may do a little better next time round. If you can do two pull-ups, well done. You have probably achieved the standard entry. If you can do five, well, it's the elite forces for you!

Women

- Hang horizontally from a gymnastics beam
- Place your hands in an overhand grip
- Extend your arms and legs
- Place your heels on a bench or similar
- Raise your body until your chest touches the beam
- Lower yourself until your arms are fully extended (don't flex the hips or knees or push off with your heels)

Keep going for as long as you can with calm, controlled movements.

Sit-ups

- Lie on your back with your hands folded behind your head
- Rest your lower legs and buttocks against a box
- Get a partner to hold down your feet
- Raise your torso using your abdominal muscles
- Touch your right knee with your left elbow
- Lower yourself
- Raise your torso and touch your left knee with your right elbow

The requirements for grade 3 are 24 reps for men, 14 reps for women, and for grade 6 they are 45 reps for men, 26 reps for women.

Push-ups

- Get face down on the floor
- Align your forefingers with the outer edges of your shoulders, fingers pointing straight ahead
- Raise your body so that your arms are fully extended
- Lower yourself until your chest and chin touch the floor
- Flex your body trunk slightly throughout the movement so as to avoid touching the floor

Keep repeating the movements for as long as you can.

Officers, Non-Commissioned Officers and Enlisted Personnel

The physical fitness tests for officers, non-commissioned officers, and enlisted personnel are classified by three test groups, A, B, and C, which consist of aerobic tests and proficiency badges, each of which is allocated a certain number of points, giving a test score. For example, completing a military pentathlon proficiency test gives a score of 4.

Test Group A

Here is a selection of the tests:

- **547yd (500m) swim:** You will need to swim 547yd (500m) in a swimming pool no less than 13.7yd (12.5m) long. You can swim with either freestroke or breaststroke.
- **12-mile (20km) cycling:** The cycling test course is a circuit with the start and finish at the same location. The course is between slightly and moderately hilly.

Test Group B proficiency badges

Military personnel can embark on a series of physically demanding proficiency badges, many of them designed for the Scandinavian snowbound environment. A passed proficiency test corresponds to a score of 4. For two or more badges a score of 6 is awarded. The tests include:

- **The Military Pentathlon Badge:** Shooting, track obstacle course, swim obstacle course, hand grenade throw, and cross-country running.
- **Military Skiing Badge:** 18.6-mile (30km) cross-country skiing with backpack and weapon.

- **Military Marching Badge:** 18.6-mile (30km) march with backpack and weapon.
- **Infantry Badge:** 7.5–9.3-mile (12–15km) cross-country running with shooting, communication, distance evaluation, and goal setting.
- **Field Sport Badge:** shooting, map reading, and orienteering.
- **Biathlon Badge:** 6.2–12-mile (10–20km) cross-country skiing with rifle shooting.
- **Nijmegen Medal:** A four-day march with daily distances of 18.6–31 miles (30–50km).

Test Group C

Test group C consists of proficiency badges and a walking test. These are:

- **Sports Badge:** Track and field, swimming, cycling, cross-country skiing, skating, walking, orienteering, throwing or weight lifting.
- **Swimming Proficiency Badge:** Swimming, underwater swimming, floating, diving, and undressing in water.
- **9.3-mile (15km) walk.**

A passed proficiency test corresponds to the minimum military physical standard, which is a score of 2.

9.3-mile (15km) walk

Recruits must walk 9.3 miles (15km) with one foot in contact with the ground at all times (so that the walk is not confused with a run). The course should be marked with signs at intervals of 3.1 and 6.2 miles (5 and 10km), preferably at 0.6-mile (1km) intervals.

Basic Officer Training Tests

These tests include a personal skills assessment based on performance in the 1.9-mile (3km) run, pull-ups, sit-ups, and push-ups (see "Military Personnel" for test descriptions). The assessment also requires the completion of a 219yd (200m) swim before and two orienteering runs after admission to basic officer training. The minimum requirement for admission to basic officer training for an officer cadet in the 1.9-mile (3km) run is:

- 14:30 minutes for men
- 15:30 minutes for women
- An average score of 4 in the three muscular fitness tests
- Completion of a 219yd (200m) swim

The corresponding requirements for a non-commissioned officer cadet in the 1.9-mile (3km) run is:

- 14 minutes for men
- 15 minutes for women,
- An average score of 4 in the three muscle fitness tests
- Completion of a 219yd (200m) swim

In addition to theory, the personal skills assessment forms the basis for a grade in physical education after admission to basic officer training. The grade in physical education can be further improved by 0.5 points by completing three of the following proficiency badges: marching, infantry, pentathlon, skiing, field sport, biathlon, swimming proficiency.

Orienteering

Recruits run on a varied orienteering course, where the basic time is calculated on the basis of the average time of 60 percent of the test results. If you want to experience the flavor of this test, contact your local orienteering club.

SPANISH ARMED FORCES

The Spanish Armed Forces provide protection for the Kingdom of Spain as well as being an active member of the North Atlantic Treaty Organisation (NATO). The Spanish Armed Forces are often engaged in global peace support and humanitarian missions. The entry requirements consist of seven different tests, which have different levels depending on the service.

Vertical Jump

Objective: To test leg power.

Requirements: A flat, hard surface and a wall or other vertical surface marked in inches to the required height. Chalk or talcum powder (for the hands).

Starting position: Stand next to the wall and raise both your arms. Mark the height you can reach.

The test: To jump as high as possible. Mark the height reached.

Rules: The test result will be the number of inches between the highest level reached while standing and the height reached when jumping. Arms can be moved, trunk flexed, knees bent, and heels lifted, but feet cannot leave the ground before making the jump. On the test day the recruit is allowed two attempts and their score will be the highest mark achieved out of the two attempts.

Push-Ups

Objective: To test arm and body muscles.

Requirements: A flat surface and a small pillow.

Starting position: Get down on the ground with your hands shoulder-width apart and your arms straight.

The test: Complete as many push-ups

Spanish Armed Forces physical fitness tests

	General entry		Marines	
	M	F	M	F
Vertical jump	13in (33cm)	11$\frac{7}{16}$in (29 cm)	16$\frac{9}{16}$in (42cm)	14$\frac{3}{16}$in (36cm)
Push-ups	9	7	18	12
55yd (50m) swim	1:22 min	1:35 min	1 min	1:08 min
55yd (50m) run	9 sec	9.9 sec	8 sec	8.8 sec
1,094yd (1,000m) run	5:10 min	6:22 min	3:55 min	4:25 min
Obstacle course	16 min	19 min	14 min	16 min

as you can, bearing in mind that the only push-ups that will be counted will be those where your chin touches the small pillow. Throughout the test, your shoulders, back, and legs should be straight.

Bear in mind: You can rest at any time during the exercise, so long as your arms remain straight. You cannot rest any part of your body on the ground during the process of the push-up, apart from your chin and toes.

55yd (50m) Swim

Objective: To assess strength and ability in water.

Requirements: A pool of the required length and a stopwatch.

The test: Stand on the side of the pool and, once the signal has been given, jump into the water and swim 55yd (50m) freestyle as fast as you can.

Bear in mind: You cannot rest either on the floor of the pool or on the sides. When you finish the first lap you can touch the wall with any part of your body and then push off with your feet for the return swim. The test will be over when you touch the wall of the pool at the moment you arrive so that the tester can see you. There is only one attempt at the test. The tester will determine at the end of the test whether all of the criteria have been fulfilled. Only one false start is allowed.

55yd (50m) Run

Objective: Measure sprinting speed.

The test: Once the signal has been given, sprint at maximum speed to the finishing tape.

Bear in mind: This is an individual event to be run at maximum pace. You can have two attempts, with a pause between each one. Only one false start is allowed for each attempt.

1,094yd (1,000m) Run

Objective: To measure overall endurance.

The test: To complete the course at maximum speed within the required time.

Obstacle Course

Objective: To measure agility, speed, and coordination.

The test: There is a test course consisting of flag markers on poles and two hurdles. The course is designed to test coordination and the ability to follow instructions clearly, as well as speed, agility, strength, and determination. Run from the right-hand side of the first set of hurdles, round to the left of the left flag, round to the right of the second hurdle, under the second hurdle from the far side. Now facing the way you came, run back to the left of the other flag, then round to the right of the first hurdle, then under the first hurdle from the far side, then straight through the middle of the flags to jump the second hurdle.

The Spanish Armed Forces also recommend a variety of training exercises so that recruits are prepared for the tests.

For the obstacle course they recommend the following preparation:

- **Sprinting trials:** Twice a week.
- **Knee raises:** Raising each knee consecutively so that your upper leg is at 90 degrees to the ground. Do three sets of ten for each knee.
- **Forward knee raises:** Do the knee raises while moving forward over a 50ft (15m) course.
- **Hurdles:** Place eight hurdles over a distance of 164ft (50m), with 20ft (6m) between them and at a height of 2.4ft (72cm, which is the height of the hurdles in the test). Three repetitions twice a week.
- **Zigzags:** Place seven cones in a straight line, with 10ft (3m) between each cone. Run through them four times.

Military personnel are encouraged to take every opportunity to build and maintain their physical fitness. A relaxed jog on the beach, such as these Spanish soldiers are taking, can loosen up the body after intensive exercise.

SWEDISH ARMED FORCES

The Swedish Armed Forces provide protection for the homeland as well as being involved in missions abroad. Before attempting the entry tests candidates are advised to work through the brochure of recommended training, which includes a variety of exercises such as step-ups, squats, heel raises, split squats, chin-ups, dips, push-ups, back lifts, diagonal lifts, sit-ups, oblique sit-ups, pelvic lifts, the plank, and deadlifts.

FM (Swedish Armed Forces) Physical Standards

These tests range from basic level tests to special physical fitness tests for certain positions. The FM Physical Fitness Standards include regular physical training, with a minimum of two training sessions per week to promote physical fitness, strength, and mobility. The plan covers individual training goals, training planning, physical training, and follow-up evaluation. The aim is to produce personnel who have sufficient capability for their roles and also improved health, well-being, and quality of life.

Field test 2,187yd (2,000m)

The test for soldiers is conducted on level ground in combat gear, including a slung weapon. The recommended surface of the test course is hard-packed gravel (or similar). The average time requirement is 12:30 minutes.

Multi-Strength Test

The Multi-Strength Test is carried out as a set of tests in the following order: push-ups, sit-ups, vertical jump, back suspension, arm suspension. The maximum time for completion of the tests is 45 minutes. You have to achieve at least the minimum level in

> THE TEST IS
> CONDUCTED ON LEVEL
> GROUND IN COMBAT
> GEAR, INCLUDING
> A WEAPON

each test (see table, page 91). The number of repetitions, height, or time exceeding the minimum level is multiplied by a coefficient, which results in a given amount of points for each subtest. The maximum number of points per subtest is 100. The requirement for passing the Multi-Strength Test is the achievement of the minimum level in all subtests.

Push-ups

- Get down on the ground with your feet hip-width apart on the ground
- Place your hands in a comfortable position
- Straighten your arms and body
- Flex your arms until the upper arms are parallel to the ground

The test cycle is completed by extending the arms back to the starting position. Complete as many push-ups as possible. The rate of push-ups is set using a metronome, which is set to 50 beats/min (25 repetitions/min).

Sit-ups

- Get into a sitting position with your arms linked, resting on your knees
- Flex your knees at 90 degrees, keeping your feet partly in contact with the floor and your gaze forward
- Lower your trunk until your shoulders reach the ground
- Raise your trunk back to the starting position to complete the test cycle
- Link your arms throughout the test movement and keep them in contact with the chest in the lower position

Your feet and buttocks should also remain in contact with the ground throughout the movement. The test should be performed rhythmically and with as many consecutive repetitions as possible between the minimum and maximum level stated for each subtest. The working speed is set using a metronome at 50 beats/min (25 repetitions/min).

Vertical jump

- Perform the test from an upright position with your legs straight and feet shoulder-width apart
- A flexible measuring tape should be attached to your waist so that it hangs down from your back to the ground
- A ruler (or similar) is taped flat to the floor

- After you have assumed the starting position with flexed legs and hips, the free end of the measuring tape should be fed in under the ruler
- Use your arms in a pendulum effect to jump straight up as high as possible with your body in a vertical position in the upper part of the position

Upon landing, the marking is read on the measuring tape at the edge of the ruler. The highest jump out of three approved jumps is recorded and used for calculating points for the test.

Back suspension

- Lie on your stomach with the edge of your hip bone level with the edge of the bench (or similar)
- Your lower legs should be anchored onto the bench immediately below the knee joint
- Your body should be horizontal and your hands linked behind the ears with the elbows away from the body
- Remain horizontal (in the starting position) for as long as possible
- This must be between the minimum and maximum suspension time
- The timing starts when you assume the starting position and stops when the measure (hung from the neck) touches the floor

- The number of seconds you remain suspended is recorded

Arm suspension

For this exercise you can get help in assuming the starting position.

- Grip the bar with an underhand grip, hands shoulder-width apart
- Keep your chin above the bar (or similar) with your gaze forward and your head in a natural position
- Your body should be suspended vertically and remain still and your chin should not touch the bar

Timing starts when the starting position is assumed and stops when your chin dips below the bar. The number of seconds you remain suspended is recorded, and must be between the minimum and maximum suspension time.

Officer Physical Fitness Tests

All of the following tests are to be carried out and passed within six months before final admission to the Officers' Program.

22yd (20m) shuttle run/bleep test

See page 166 for a full description of the bleep test. The highest achieved level and shuttle is recorded as the test score.

Multi-Strength Test points table

Test	Min	Max	Points
Push-ups	8	28	5 points/rep
Sit-ups	10	60	2 points/rep
Vertical jump	11^{13}/₁₆in (30cm)	19^{11}/₁₆in (50cm)	5 points/cm
Back suspension	60 sec	160 sec	1 point/sec
Arm suspension	15 sec	65 sec	2 points/sec

Swimming 437yd (400m)

This test starts when you either dive or jump (your head must go under the surface of the water) into a 27 or 55yd (25 or 50m) swimming pool with a water temperature of at least 68°F (20°C) and a pool depth of at least 5.7ft (1.75m) at the starting point. The swimming test is a distance swim of 437yd (400m) without rest. You are not allowed to touch the pool floor or the pool edge at the long sides or the track lines in the pool. The pool edge at the short sides can only be touched with the hands and feet during the turning movement. Hanging on the edge is not permitted. Any swimming style may be used, and it may be changed during the test.

The Swedish Armed Forces suggest the following swimming training exercises:

Training Exercise 1

- Start sitting on the side of the pool
- Get into the water and swim to the bottom of the pool
- Swim back to the side of the pool in a different place
- With your back to the wall of the pool, pull yourself up onto the side
- Get back in the water and swim to the bottom before returning to the side
- Repeat

Training Exercise 2

- Dive into the water
- Swim to the other side of the pool
- Get out and do ten push-ups or sit-ups

ROYAL AUSTRALIAN NAVY

As the senior service in the Australian Defense Force, the Royal Australian Navy (RAN) has a busy time protecting the coastline of the world's largest island country. Although there is a general entry test for the service, the swimming component is particularly important as it leads to RAN Sea Familiarization Training. All RAN recruits must pass the RAN Physical Fitness Test, which is conducted in the first week of training.

RAN Physical Fitness Test Requirements

In order to pass, recruits need to reach the required standard in the three parts of the test listed below. That is good news because if you attempt the test and pass, it will show you have achieved a high level of strength as well as aerobic fitness.

- Military push-ups or flexed-arm hang (push-ups conducted at a 2-second cadence)
- Military sit-ups (sit-ups conducted at a 3-second cadence)
- A 1.5-mile (2.4km) run

Swim Test

All members of the RAN are also required to undertake the RAN Swim Test. Passing the swim test is a requirement in the RAN in order to graduate from Recruit School and also to go on to Safety of Life at Sea Training, part of the Sea Familiarisation Training. For the test, recruits wear overalls and swim in any manner of their choosing. This is important because it reflects a real-life situation, such as an "abandon ship" scenario where you would be likely to have to swim for your life fully clothed.

RAN Physical Fitness Test requirements

	Less than 35 years		35–44 years		45–54 years		55 plus	
	M	F	M	F	M	F	M	F
Push-ups	25 reps	25 reps	20 reps	7 reps	6 reps	3 reps	6 reps	3 reps
Flexed-arm hang	25 sec	25 sec	20 sec	20 sec	15 sec	15 sec	10 sec	10 sec
Sit-ups	25 reps	25 reps	20 reps	20 reps	15 reps	15 reps	10 reps	10 reps
1.5-mile (2.4km) run	13 min	13 min	15 min	19 min	17 min	19 min	19 min	21 min
547yd (500m) swim (min)	12:30 min	12:30 min	13:30 min	14:30 min	14:30 min	15:30 min	15:30 min	16:30 min
Bleep test	7.4	7.4	6.10	6.2	6.4	5.4	5.9	5.0

> # IT IS RECOMMENDED THAT RECRUITS HAVE SWIMMING TRAINING BEFORE THEY START THE COURSE

The RAN Swim Test consists of:
- 10ft (3m) safety jump from a platform
- 33ft (10m) underwater swim (body fully submerged under water)
- 55yd (50m) swim using survival strokes only (breaststroke, back scull, or sidestroke)
- 15 minutes treading water in overalls

It is highly recommended that recruits have swimming training before they start the course.

RAN Naval Clearance Diver and Naval Reserve Diver applicants have different Pre-Entry Fitness Assessment requirements. This is because they have a particularly demanding role which not only involves swimming long distances and at considerable depth, often with heavy equipment, but also carrying out special forces duties as part of a Tactical Assault Group (TAG). Requirements are:
- 6 chin-ups
- 30 push-ups
- 25 sit-ups
- 10.1 shuttle run score

AUSTRALIAN DEFENSE FORCE PERSONAL FITNESS ASSESSMENTS

The Australian Defense Force requires its members to maintain a high standard of physical fitness. A variety of activities have been devised to help them reach the required level of fitness. Part of the ongoing fitness regime is organized sport, in which all members of the Defense Force are encouraged to take part when their training program allows it.

Navy

The PFA for Navy entry consists of push-ups, sit-ups, and a shuttle run.

Male requirement: 15 push-ups, 20 sit-ups (feet held), 6.1 shuttle run score.

Female requirement: 6 push-ups, 20 sit-ups (feet held), 6.1 shuttle run score.

The only exceptions are Navy Clearance Diver and Naval Reserve Diver applicants, who must pass the PFA at the following standards: 6 heaves (chin-ups), 30 push-ups, 25 sit-ups, and a 10.1 shuttle run score.

Army

The PFA for Navy entry consists of push-ups, sit-ups, and a shuttle run.

Male requirement: 15 push-ups, 45 sit-ups, 7.5 shuttle run score

Female requirement: 8 push-ups, 45 sit-ups, 7.5 shuttle run score

For Special Forces Direct Recruiting Scheme (SFDRS) candidates (male only), the PFA standards are 30 push-ups, 60 sit-ups, and 10.1 shuttle run score.

Australian soldiers participate in a fire and movement exercise, which is part of a comprehensive series of fitness tests.

Air Force

The PFA for Air Force entry consists of push-ups, sit-ups, and a shuttle run.

Male requirement: 10 push-ups, 20 sit-ups (feet held), 6.5 shuttle run score

Female requirement: 4 push-ups, 20 sit-ups (feet held), 6.5 shuttle run score

For applicants over the age of 55 the following standards will be required:

Male requirement: 5 push-ups, 20 sit-ups (feet held), 6.5 shuttle run score

Female requirement: 3 push-ups, 20 sit-ups (feet held), 6.5 shuttle run score

The only exceptions are Ground Defense Officer and Airfield Defense Guard applicants, who must pass the PFA at the following standards: 15 push-ups, 45 sit-ups, 7.5 shuttle run score.

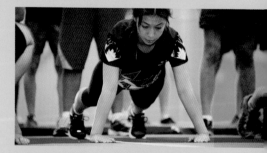

BRITISH ROYAL NAVY

The Royal Navy is the senior service in the British Armed Forces and carries out a wide range of missions both in home waters and across the globe. Swimming is obviously an important part of a naval entry test. The general entry test includes a realistic "abandon ship" scenario assessment, whereas the tests for the Royal Navy Mine Clearance Diver (see page 122) are geared toward endurance and strength.

The UK Royal Navy runs a Naval Service Pre-Joining Fitness Test which includes the following minimum standards:

- **1.5-mile (2.4km) run:** On a treadmill. To be completed by men (age under 24) in 11:09 minutes and by women in 13:10 minutes
- **Push-ups:** 23 for men and 17 for women
- **Sit-ups:** 39 for men and 29 for women
- **Shuttle run:** 5 × 60yd (55m) to be completed in 59 seconds for men and 72 seconds for women

As it is the Navy, there is no surprise that there is also a swimming test. The recruits have to jump into a pool wearing overalls, tread water for 2 minutes and then swim 55yd (50m) before climbing out at the end. This, of course, is done under close supervision; you should not attempt this part of the test alone.

The Royal Navy recommend an eight-week fitness training program for potential recruits. Warming up and stretching are seen as essential components in the program. The fitness program includes both cardiovascular and anaerobic exercises such as running,

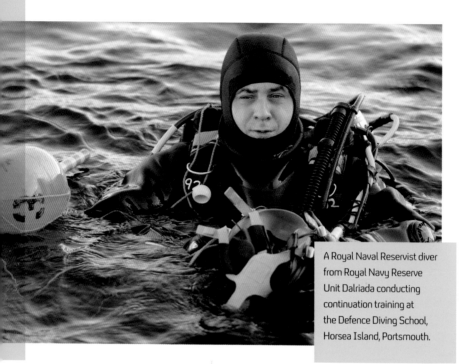

A Royal Naval Reservist diver from Royal Navy Reserve Unit Dalriada conducting continuation training at the Defence Diving School, Horsea Island, Portsmouth.

swimming, and strength training on a gradually incremental basis. Upper body and abdominal exercises include push-ups, trunk curls, dorsal raises, and the plank position.

The Navy emphasise that the fitness requirements in the tests are minimum standards and that recruits should aim to achieve the run within the timing parameters and also aim to complete more repetitions of upper-body exercises than those specified.

THE GENERAL ENTRY TEST INCLUDES A REALISTIC "ABANDON SHIP" SCENARIO ASSESSMENT

US NAVY

From around the time of the Second World War (1939–45), the United States Navy took over from the British Royal Navy as the world's largest and most powerful naval force. It is divided into the Pacific Fleet, the Atlantic Fleet, Naval Forces Europe, and Central Command. Its major role is the defense of the United States, seaborne support of other US armed forces and NATO allies, as well as a wide range of strategic, peace support, and humanitarian operations.

US Navy Physical Fitness Test

This test consists of:
- **1.5-mile (2.4km) run:** In optimum time
- **Sit-ups:** Maximum achievable in 2 minutes
- **Push-ups:** Maximum number achievable in 2 minutes

The final PFT score is made up of an average of the scores for each event.

The Card Series

Fitness is given special priority in the US Navy for one good reason. If you are at sea, it can be difficult to go for a long run or a cycle ride or swim in a full-size pool. Navy personnel therefore need to be ingenious about maintaining their fitness so that they can be ready for action at any time.

The US Navy have put together an elaborate fitness training program known as the card series. This is designed to provide fitness advice for a variety of different types of naval vessel. For example, the fitness challenges faced by

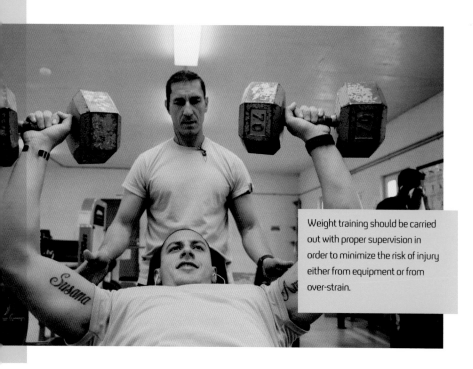

Weight training should be carried out with proper supervision in order to minimize the risk of injury either from equipment or from over-strain.

the crew of a submarine are different from those on an aircraft carrier. For each series (e.g. Submarine Series or Large Deck Series) there are three levels of training, each of which is broken down into four stages. It is highly recommended that sailors work up through the stages, only moving on to the next level once they have achieved mastery of the level they are on.

The card fitness series is designed to fit into a sailor's working schedule and therefore needs to be adaptable. Each of the fitness programs has three different timings: Short (30 minutes), Medium (45 minutes), and Long (60 minutes). Each training session consists of five separate components:

1. Pillar Preparation (hips, torso, and shoulders)
2. Movement
3. Strength
4. Cardiovascular
5. Recovery

BRITISH ROYAL AIR FORCE

Officially formed in 1918 as a development of the Royal Flying Corps, the Royal Air Force (RAF) is the world's first independent air force. Today it is tasked with the defense of the United Kingdom, while also providing strategic support for the other armed services. It operates globally and is able to provide support for peace and humanitarian missions abroad.

The RAF has three kinds of test:

1. Selection Fitness Test
2. Pre-Joining Fitness Test
3. Pre-Recruit Training Course

The Pre-Joining Fitness Test includes:

- A 1.5-mile (2.4km) run to be completed in 11:11 minutes for men and 13:23 minutes for women (age 17–29)
- 20 push-ups for men and 10 for women (age 17–29)
- 35 sit-ups for men and 32 for women (age 17–29)

Also part of the package is the multi-stage fitness test (MSFT), or bleep test: the pass score for men is 9.10 and for women 7.02. In addition, those over 18 must have a Body Mass Index (BMI) of between 18 and 28.2.

> THE RAF OPERATES GLOBALLY, PROVIDING SUPPORT FOR PEACE AND HUMANITARIAN MISSIONS ABROAD

Selection Fitness Test requirements

Age	1.5-mile (2.4km) run (minutes)		Multi-stage fitness test		Push-ups		Sit-ups	
	M	F	M	F	M	F	M	F
15–16	11:39	13:54	9.03	6.07	20	10	35	32
17–29	11:11	13:23	9.1	7.02	20	10	35	32
30–34	11:36	13:47	9.04	6.08	19	9	32	29
35–39	12:00	14:13	8.09	6.04	18	8	29	26
40–44	12:26	14:48	8.03	5.08	17	7	26	23
45–49	12:54	15:19	7.07	5.04	16	6	23	20
50–54	13:27	15:53	7.01	4.09	15	5	20	17

Pre-Joining Fitness Test requirements

Age	1.5-mile (2.4km) run (minutes) 100% Pass		Push-ups 100% Pass		Sit-ups 100% Pass	
	M	F	M	F	M	F
15–16	11:39	13:54	20	10	35	32
17–29	11:11	13:23	20	10	35	32
30–34	11:36	13:47	19	9	32	29
35–39	12:00	14:13	18	8	29	26
40–44	12:26	14:48	17	7	26	23

Pre-Recruit Training Course requirements

Age	Multi-stage fitness test 100% Pass		Push-ups 100% Pass		Sit-ups 100% Pass	
	M	F	M	F	M	F
15–16	9.03	6.07	20	10	35	32
17–29	9.1	7.02	20	10	35	32
30–34	9.04	6.08	19	9	32	29
35–39	8.09	6.04	18	8	29	26
40–44	8.03	5.08	17	7	26	23

US AIR FORCE

The US Air Force is tasked with the defense of the United States and is also capable of carrying out proportionate offensive missions on a global scale. The US Air Force often works in cooperation with other services, such as naval or military special forces, in carrying out close air support and ground attack missions. The USAF's heavy-lift capacity enables it to carry out valuable humanitarian relief operations.

To join the USAF the recruit needs to be between 17 and 39 years old and must pass the Armed Services Vocational Aptitude Battery (ASVAB), which covers areas such as mathematical skills and verbal reasoning. Candidates then visit a Military Entrance Processing Station (MEPS) where they undergo various tests. The United States Air Force Fitness Assessment (FA) is designed to test overall fitness, including muscular strength and cardiovascular fitness. The assessment includes:

1. Height and weight measurement (for record only).

2. Abdominal circumference measurement (measurement taken around the waist just above the hip bone). Maximum measurement 39in (99cm); target 37in (94cm) or lower.

3. Number of push-ups in 1 minute (minimum requirement 27; target 39 or better).

4. Number of sit-ups in 1 minute (minimum requirement 39; target 42 or better).

5. 1.5-mile (2.4km) run in best time (minimum requirement 13:37–14 minutes; target 12:54–13:14 minutes or better).

Basic military training graduation requirements

Males	2-mile (3.2km) run		1.5-mile (2.4km) run		Push-ups		Sit-ups		Pull-ups	
	M	F	M	F	M	F	M	F	M	F
Minimum standard	16:45 min	19:45 min	11:57 min	13:56 min	45	27	50	50	0	0
Honor graduate standard	14:15 min	16:00 min	8:55 min	11:33 min	62	37	70	60	4	2
Highest standard	13:30 min	15:00 min	8:08 min	10:55 min	75	40	80	75	10	5

Recruits can earn up to 100 points and the minimum score is 75. As with all fitness tests, it is highly recommended that you not only meet but surpass the fitness standard.

Preparation is key, whether it is a fitness test or giving a presentation. Your confidence will be transformed if you know deep down that you are well prepared and that you can do it within the allocated time. Real recruits also need to be confident that they have the basic fitness that will get them through Basic Military Training.

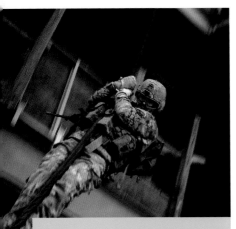

Physical strength and coordination are important when carrying out dangerous maneuvers such as fast-roping, here being practiced from a training tower by an Air Force Combat Control trainee.

INDIAN AIR FORCE

The Indian Air Force (IAF) was established in 1932 with officers trained by the British Royal Air Force. It fought against the Japanese in Burma during the Second World War and since then has been involved in four wars. Its primary duty is the protection of Indian air space. It is also regularly involved in United Nations Peacekeeping Missions and disaster relief, including the Tsunami of 2004.

The Indian Air Force is divided into five operational commands and two functional commands. Officer training is based at the Air Force Academy at Dundigul, near Hyderabad. To become an officer in the IAF, candidates must be under 23 years old at the time of application. After completion of training, a candidate is commissioned as a Flying Officer.

The Test

All candidates for the Indian Air Force must pass the Physical Fitness Test (PFT) before moving on with further training. The PFT consists of:

- A 1-mile (1.6km) run to be completed within 8 minutes
- The IAF (Security) trade applicants must complete a 1.5-mile (2.4km) run and a 3.1-mile (5km) run in 15 minutes and 30 minutes respectively

Garud Commando Force

The Garud Commando Force is the special operations force of the IAF and consists of about 1,500 personnel organized into fifteen flights, under a Flight Officer. The Garud Commando Force carries out combat search and rescue (CSR), suppression of enemy air defense (SEAD), and other air support missions. Candidates for the Garud Commando Force are selected from Airmen Selection Centres, where they need to show exceptional potential.

Training for the Garud Commando Force includes 72 weeks' basic training, which begins at Garud Regimental Training Centre at Hindon, Ghaziabad. It takes about three years to qualify as a Garud Commando. The next stage of training is done with the Special Group of Special Frontier Force, including army and paramilitary forces. They then move on to Parachute Training School (PTS) at Agra for the basic airborne phase. Here they are trained alongside paratroopers of the Indian Army.

Recruits then move on to specialized training for jungle, snow survival, demolitions, advanced driving skills, anti-hijack and counter-insurgency training, and specialized weapon handling.

Training establishments for this phase include the Indian Navy diving school, Army Counter Insurgency and Jungle Warfare School (CIJWS), and an attachment to the Indian Army Special Forces.

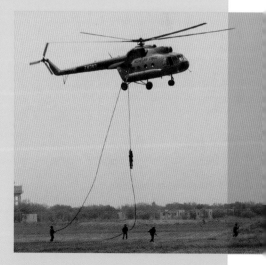

BRITISH ARMY PARACHUTE REGIMENT

The Parachute Regiment is an elite force in the British Army and corresponds to the Royal Marines in the Royal Navy. It forms a spearhead force that can be rapidly deployed by air, taking its essential equipment with it and holding the area until larger forces arrive. Members of the First Battalion (1 Para) are incorporated into the UK Special Forces Support Group, where they provide operational support for special forces units such as the Special Air Service (SAS).

The British Parachute Regiment Entrance Fitness Test includes:

- 1.5-mile (2.4km) run between 9:30 and 9:40 minutes
- A 4-mile (6.4km) familiarization run
- 50 push-ups in 2 minutes
- 50 sit-ups in 2 minutes
- 7 pull-ups

Parachute Regiment's P Company Selection Course

To get into the Pathfinder Platoon the recruit first needs to pass the Parachute Regiment's P Company Selection Course. First they should attend P Company Preparation Course. This lasts for six weekends over a 12-week period and is designed to improve the candidate's physical fitness, stamina, and robustness. The various exercises include running, marching, and carrying weighted backpacks over undulating terrain. There are seven test events over a four and a half day period. Six are scored while one (the Trainasium) is a straight pass/fail. Each event is designed to assess their physical fitness, mental robustness, and determination. Recruits need to display self-discipline and motivation throughout in order to pass the course.

10-Mile March: A 10-mile (16km) march is conducted as a squad, over undulating terrain with each candidate carrying a bergan (backpack). The event is a straight pass/fail.

Log Race: This is a team event with 8 candidates carrying a 132lb (60kg) log a distance of 1.9 miles (3km) over undulating terrain.

2-Mile March: The 2-mile (3.2km) march is conducted over undulating terrain with each individual carrying a bergan weighing 35lb (16kg), plus water and a weapon. They also wear a helmet and combat jacket. The time required is under 19 minutes.

Steeplechase: This is an individual test with candidates running against the clock over a 1.9-mile (3km) cross-country course. The course features a number of water obstacles. Having completed the cross-country element, candidates must negotiate an assault course to complete the test and get within 19 minutes.

Milling: This consists of 60 seconds of controlled physical aggression against an opponent of similar height and weight.

Stretcher Race: The final event of P Company. Teams of 16 men carry a 175lb (79kg) stretcher over a distance of 5 miles (8km). No more than four men carry the stretcher at any time. Individuals wear webbing and carry a weapon.

THE TRAINASIUM

The Trainasium is a 60ft (18m) high aerial confidence course where recruits have to overcome their fear of heights while carrying out various physical tasks. These include walking along parallel steel bars, running on moving surfaces (simulating the movement of a plane), swinging from ropes, and jumping across open spaces at height. All of the tasks have to be performed instantly and with confidence, otherwise it is a straight fail. There are no points on the Trainasium; a recruit can either do it or they can't. If they cannot do it at 60ft (18m), they will not be able to jump out of a plane at 800ft (244m).

AUSTRALIAN SPECIAL FORCES

All applicants for the Australian Special Forces must pass the Special Forces Pre-Fitness Assessment (PFA). It is set at a higher standard than the test for the Australian Army. The PFA is the minimum standard for enlistment as a potential commando candidate. A much higher level of physical fitness is required to complete the Commando Selection and Training Course. Regular participation in sports, fitness activities, or outdoor pursuits is excellent ground work for commando entry.

Special Forces PFA

The test consists of:

- Bleep test (shuttle run) to level 10.1
- 30 push-ups (two-minute time limit)
- 60 sit-ups

Special Forces Screen Test

In order to confirm that candidates have the right level of commitment and motivation and that they are capable of enduring the demands of the Commando Selection and Training Course, their aptitude is tested in the Special Forces Screen Test. The real test lasts about 7 hours and includes a range of challenging physical assessments. However, if you want to experience some of the flavor of the assessment, take a pick from some of the example test disciplines below. For special forces entry there is no minimum or maximum standard; recruits are measured against the overall standard of their group. So the sky's the limit!

- **Push-ups (cadence):** No further explanation needed. Do as many as you can and then more.

- **Chin-ups (cadence):** Same as above.

- **Vertec (vertical leap):** You can read more about how to do a vertical leap in Part Three of this book. The good news is that without exhausting yourself too much, you can gain some extra brownie points by getting your technique right. A good way to practice for the Vertec is to do plenty of squats.

- **Sit-up test:** Do as many as you can.

- **Yo-Yo intermittent recovery test:** This is a bleep test (see page 166) with a difference. The test is often used to train and test footballers, who need to sprint and recover quickly. Special forces also need to move fast and recover quickly as part of their job. Like the bleep test, you need to run between two points within the time that a beep sounds. With the recovery test, after you reach the point you then walk a few meters further as part of the recovery, walk round a cone, and back to the start before the beep starts you off on your next run. This test will assess your ability to perform high-intensity exercise.

- **Pack march:** A distance of 3 miles (5km) carrying 88lb (40kg). Load up your backpack and off you go.

Remember to take plenty of water with you and wear a good pair of boots that will provide support with the extra weight.

- **Swim test:** Tread water for 2 minutes before swimming 437yd (400m) in Disruptive Pattern Combat Uniform (DPCU). This part of the test is here for information purposes only: it is not recommended that you attempt to swim in clothing unless you are on a specific course with safety personnel present.

The standard in the Special Forces Screening Test is the individual performance of each candidate against the rest. At the test, a Selection Advisory Committee decides whether candidates have the potential for service in Special Forces and whether they should go on to the Commando Selection and Training Course. This decision takes into account overall performance at recruit training, infantry training, and the Accelerated Infantry Training program, as well as the results from the Special Forces Screen Test.

JAEGERKORPSET

Based at Aalborg in Northern Jutland, the Jaegerkorpset (Danish Ranger Force) is an elite unit of about 100 operators with a big reputation in reconnaissance and counter-terrorism. It was formed in 1961, based on the models of the British Special Air Service (SAS) and US Rangers, and has expertise in long-range reconnaissance patrols (LRRP). The Jaegerkorpset sometimes work with the Danish special police unit Aktions Styrken on counter-terrorist missions. Comprehensive training includes High Altitude High Opening (HAHO) parachute drops and the British Armed Forces often provide helicopters for Jaegerkorpset insertions.

Danish Defence Recruitment Test

To join the elite Danish Ranger Force, the Jaegerkorpset, the recruit will need first to pass the basic Danish Defence Recruitment Test and then the commando course entry requirements. To enter the Jaegerkorpset patrol course recruits need to pass the following tests:

Marching

March 18.6 miles (30km) wearing kit and carrying equipment weighing about 66lb (30kg), to be completed in a maximum of 6 hours.

Swimming

This takes place at the start of the patrol course, and the candidate wears trunks and goggles.

- 55yd (50m) freestyle in a maximum of 50 seconds
- 328yd (300m) breaststroke in a maximum of 7:30 minutes
- 1,094yd (1,000m) breaststroke in a maximum of 25 minutes
- 27yd (25m) underwater swimming
- Diving from a height of 10ft (3m)

Overall physical capacity test

Course	Yo-Yo Endurance test	Lunges	Dips	Chin-ups	Core plank	Deadlifts
Introductory Course II	No test but there is a check on current level of fitness					
Introductory Course II	11.9 = K-tal 5.0	40 reps 45lb (20kg)	8 reps	8 reps	90 sec 22lb (10kg)	6 reps 154lb (70kg)
Introductory Course III	12.5 = K-tal 52.3	40 reps 66lb (30kg)	5 reps 11lb (5kg)	5 reps 11lb (5kg)	90 sec 22lb (10kg)	6 reps 154lb (70kg)
Patrol course	12. 12 = K-tal 54.3	40 reps 88lb (40kg)	8 reps 11lb (5kg)	8 reps 11lb (5kg)	120 sec 33lb (15kg)	8 reps 176lb (80kg)

Hunter Course fitness requirements

Course	Yo-Yo Endurance test	Lunges Max 2 min	Dips Max 1 min	Chin-ups Max 1 min	Core plank Max 2 min	Deadlifts Max 1 min
JGASPKUR	12:12 = K-tal 54.3	40 reps 88lb (40kg)	8 reps 11lb (5kg)	8 reps 11lb (5kg)	120 sec 33lb (15kg)	8 reps 176lb (80kg)
Character	Physical requirements	40 reps 110lb (50kg)	8 reps 22lb (10kg)	8 reps 22lb (10kg)	120 sec 45lb (20kg)	8 reps 220lb (100kg)

Hunter Course Fitness Requirements

Marching
March 31 miles (50km) wearing kit and carrying equipment weighing about 66lb (30kg), to be completed within 12 hours.

Swimming
For the swim test the recruit should wear swimming trunks and goggles. The test includes the following challenges:

- Swim 55yd (50m) freestyle in a maximum of 50 seconds
- Swim 328yd (300m) breaststroke in a maximum of 7:30 minutes
- Swim 1,094yd (1,000m) breaststroke in a maximum of 25 minutes
- Swim 27yd (25m) underwater
- Diving from 10ft (3m)

FRENCH FOREIGN LEGION

The French Foreign Legion is one of the most famous regiments in the world. More often than not, when there is a real crisis, the French State will call on the Legion to sort it out. One of the unusual characteristics of the Legion is that it will take recruits who are not French nationals, though they have to swear allegiance to the French State.

Because the French Foreign Legion is made up of individuals from a number of different nations, special emphasis is placed on building an *esprit de corps*. One of the ways that this is achieved is through tough physical training. As part of their basic training, legionnaires need to complete a 40–43-mile (65–70km) march in full kit. The standard entry test for the French Foreign Legion is relatively simple, though it includes the infamous bleep test (see page 166):

- Three pull-ups from a static position with arms extended, returning to the previous position after each pull-up
- The bleep test to test VO_2 max
- Rope climbing: Climb to the top of the rope in the correct manner
- A 12-minute run in your best possible time (the minimum standard is 3,062yd/2,800m in the time allocated)

The aim of the exercises is to achieve the highest possible score. The real fun starts once recruits are signed up to the Legion.

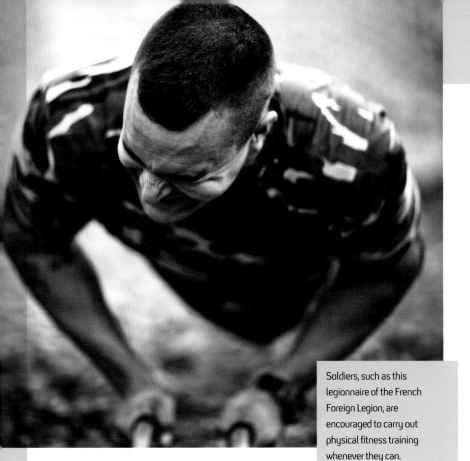

Soldiers, such as this legionnaire of the French Foreign Legion, are encouraged to carry out physical fitness training whenever they can.

FUSILIER MARINS (FRENCH COMMANDO)

Entry into the French Commandos requires high levels of physical fitness, as well as psychological balance. There is a week-long evaluation course which includes:

☑ *A VO$_2$ max test for endurance*
☑ *Rope climbing using both arms and legs*

☑ *A 219yd (200m) breaststroke swim, with 6.5ft (2m) underwater*

☑ *15 push-ups*
☑ *15 pull-ups*
☑ *40 sit-ups*

KOMMANDO SPEZIALKRAFTE

The Kommando Spezialkrafte (KSK) is a special forces regiment in the German Armed Forces, or Bundeswehr. It comes under the command of the Division Spezielle Operationen (Special Operations Division, DSO). It was set up in 1996 to supplement the work of the established Grenzschutzgruppe 9 (GSG-9). The main difference between the KSK and the GSG-9 is that the KSK is a military unit, similar to the British SAS, on which it is largely modeled, and US Delta Force.

The KSK is divided into specialist units which include:

- Paratroops
- Amphibious
- Mountain
- Snipers

Each unit is then subdivided into squads of four men, each of which will have their own specialism within the squad:

- Weapons expert
- Breacher (for forced entries)
- Radio operator
- Medic

Aptitude Test Part 1 (EFV 1)

This is an initial test of potential as a commando. The tests assess basic fitness, teamwork, and ability and willingness to learn. It lasts one week. In the Physical Fitness Test (PFT), recruits must score at least three points in each discipline:

- 547yd (500m) swim in under 15 minutes
- Five pull-ups
- Completion of the obstacle course in combat clothing, helmet, and gloves in under 1:40 hours

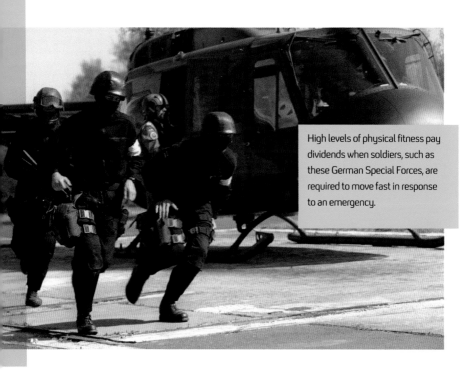

High levels of physical fitness pay dividends when soldiers, such as these German Special Forces, are required to move fast in response to an emergency.

Unlike many special forces units, entrance to the KSK is also open to civilians. Before enlisting for the KSK, recruits undergo a Long Range Surveillance course that lasts 18 months.

Initial selection consists of a three-week training course to test physical and mental attitude and strength, followed by a three-month endurance phase. This includes a 62-mile (100km) forced march carrying a backpack and other equipment, a 90-hour cross-country run, and a three-week combat survival course.

After these stages have been completed, recruits move on to two to three years of training with the KSK, including specialist training in desert, jungle, urban, amphibious, arctic, and mountain warfare, along with counter-terrorism training.

NEW ZEALAND SPECIAL AIR SERVICE

New Zealand's main special operations force is the New Zealand Special Air Service (NZSAS). The original British Special Air Service regiment (SAS), founded in 1941, was developed from the Long Range Desert Group, which included many New Zealanders. The New Zealand SAS was awarded a US Presidential Citation for its work supporting Allied operations in Afghanistan.

The SAS is divided into A and B Squadrons, which carry out the full spectrum of special forces duties, and D Squadron, which is designated specifically for counter-terrorism activities. In order to be eligible to join the NZSAS candidates need to successfully complete all of the fitness tests in the New Zealand Army to NZSAS standard. Recruits are then sent on a three-day course of open-country navigation while carrying a 77lb (35kg) pack and rifle. They are allowed a minimum allocation of food and sleep.

On the fifth day of the selection course, recruits enter the "Exercise Von Tempsky." The recruits must march in either a swamp or sand dunes while carrying rifles and alternately one or two 5.3-gallon (20l) jerricans and a 77lb (35kg) pack. In the final exercise recruits must complete a 37-mile (60km) endurance march, carrying a 77lb (35kg) pack, web gear, and rifle, in under 20 hours. Officers undergo an additional two days of selection, which includes leadership skills.

RECRUITS ARE SENT ON A 3-DAY OPEN-COUNTRY NAVIGATION COURSE

Fitness Requirements

- Pass the G1 fitness test (see below)
- Pass 4-hour endurance-based fitness tests

The NZSAS look for recruits who can operate as part of small teams in very tough conditions and who can also operate and survive on their own. This requires personality and mental qualities of endurance and initiative. It also requires a high level of physical fitness.

To get underway for selection, candidates have to pass an RFL(G1), which consists of the following:

- 8 pull-ups with an overhand grip
- 30 push-ups
- 66 sit-ups
- 1.5-mile (2.4km) run in under 10 minutes

Following this, recruits take an NZSAS Battle Endurance Test (BET):

- 5-mile (8km) walk to be completed within 72 minutes, carrying a pack and rifle with a total weight of 77lb (35kg)
- 16yd (15m) body drag
- 109yd (100m) Fireman's Carry
- Climb over a 6ft (1.8m) wall
- Complete a 16ft (5m) rope climb

The NZSAS swim test is carried out wearing military trousers and shirt and consists of the following elements:

- Treading water for 3 minutes
- Conducting a 33yd (30m) unassisted tow
- Swimming 219yd (200m) with either freestyle or breaststroke
- Swimming 16yd (15m) underwater and recovering two objects

GRUPA REAGOWANIA OPERACYJNO MOBILNEGO

The Grupa Reagowania Operacyjno Mobilnego (GROM) is the top special forces unit in Poland. The unit is about 250 strong and, unusually for a special forces unit, it also recruits women for intelligence gathering and surveillance operations. About 70 percent of GROM unit operators have advanced medical training.

General Physical Fitness Requirements

This special forces unit demands the highest levels of physical fitness and mental aptitude, though at the selection phase the main purpose is to recognize potential. The extent of your physical fitness will be seen as an indication of your attitude.

- **Pull-ups:** 16 (very good); 14 (good); 10 (satisfactory)
- **Push-ups:** 75 (very good); 70 (good); 65 (satisfactory)
- **Sit-ups:** (over a period of 2 minutes) 75 (very good); 70 (good); 65 (satisfactory)
- **Rope climb:** (to 18.4ft/5.6m): 7 seconds (very good); 9 seconds (good); 12 seconds (satisfactory)
- **10 × 11yd (10m) run:** 29.2 seconds (very good); 30.2 seconds (good); 31.2 (satisfactory)
- **1.9-mile (3km) run:** 12 minutes (very good); 13 minutes (good); 13:30 minutes (satisfactory)
- **55yd (50m) swim:** 45 seconds (very good); 55 seconds (good); 1.05 seconds (satisfactory)
- **Underwater swim:** 27yd (25m, very good); 16yd (15m, good); 11yd (10m, satisfactory)

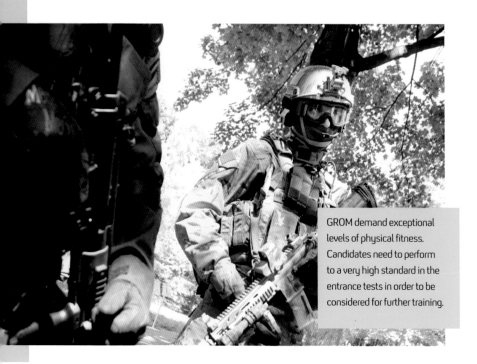

GROM demand exceptional levels of physical fitness. Candidates need to perform to a very high standard in the entrance tests in order to be considered for further training.

GROM comes under Polish Special Operations Command, or Centrum Operacji Specjalnych (COS-DKWS). There are a number of other special forces units under this command.

The oldest special forces unit is Jednostka Wojskowa Komandosov (JWK), which has similar entrance requirements and fitness standards to GROM.

GROM TASKS

1. Counter-terrorism
2. Non-combat evacuation
3. Special reconnaissance
4. Direct action
5. Military support
6. Unconventional warfare
7. Combat search and rescue

ROYAL AUSTRALIAN NAVY CLEARANCE DIVERS

One of the most demanding jobs in the Royal Australian Navy is that of Clearance Diver (CD). A CD has to dive to a depth of 177ft (54m) to check for and make safe unexploded devices. They must be exceptionally fit in order to swim long distances against powerful currents, carrying heavy equipment, often in very cold conditions.

Physical Entrance Requirements

Not only do recruits have to pass an initial fitness test, but also a Clearance Diving Acceptance (CDA) test. They undergo tough physical training throughout their careers. If you have ambitions to achieve exceptional levels in swimming either for competitions such as triathlons or for sport diving, you may want to measure yourself against these tests.

Recruits taking the CDA test have to pass a thorough medical assessment. Anyone with an illness or condition that may affect breathing ability, such as asthma or a lung condition, will not be passed. Before enlistment, the recruit also needs to pass a Physical Fitness Assessment (PFA). The PFA for CDs is set higher than the general entry requirements for the Navy. To match this test you must be able to complete:

- 6 heaves
- 30 push-ups
- 25 sit-ups
- Bleep test to level 10.1

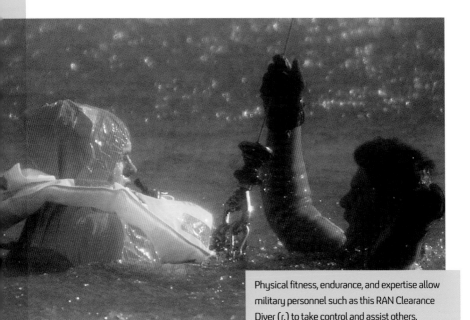

Physical fitness, endurance, and expertise allow military personnel such as this RAN Clearance Diver (r.) to take control and assist others.

Heaves/Chin-Ups

The heave/chin-up mirrors the practical requirement of CD divers to pull themselves and their equipment out of the water. The chin-ups are conducted with a pronated (overhand) grip.

Start position: Grasp the bar with your hands facing forward (pronated overhand grip), your body fully extended to a hanging position with the feet free of the ground (not crossed). You cannot change your hand position during the activity.

Pull your body upward with your arms until your chin is over the bar/beam, then lower yourself until your elbows are fully extended and your body is in the hanging position. This comprises one repetition.

You can use slight kicking motions provided that your knees do not rise above your waist and you remain vertical. Do not cross your feet at any time. An assistant can help prevent your body from swinging by extending an arm in front of you at knee height. You must complete each repetition for it to be counted. You can only rest in the starting position and without dismounting or the aid of a support.

BRITISH ROYAL NAVY MINE CLEARANCE DIVERS

Mine Clearance Divers are part of the Royal Navy. They work in great secrecy to clear mines and to prepare the area for planned amphibious landings. Mine clearance divers often have to work in very cold conditions with strong currents, usually in darkness so as to avoid detection. They need to be able to carry all their equipment and enter and leave the water unseen. Working in silence in the depths of the oceans or in estuaries and rivers, their vital work often goes unreported.

A Mine Clearance Diver usually works as part of a close-knit team of five or six divers, based either on shore or on board a Royal Navy mine countermeasures (MCM) vessel. The main task of a Mine Clearance Diver is to identify mines and other explosives, whether in shallow water or attached to the hull of a ship, and neutralize them. The job can involve using heavy equipment such as pneumatic drills at great depth. They may also need to carry out repair work on the ship's propeller or hull. Apart from being highly skilled, the role of a Mine Clearance Diver also demands very high levels of physical fitness.

The description of the diving tests here are for information purposes. Any diving related activity can only be performed in the context of professional training. Recommended build-up to fitness tests should take between six and eight weeks. First candidates need a pre-joining medical, a diving medical, an eye test, and must pass the Pre-Joining Fitness Test (PJFT), which consists of a 1.5-mile (2.4km) run on a treadmill set to a 2-degree incline. The run should be completed in under 10:30 minutes.

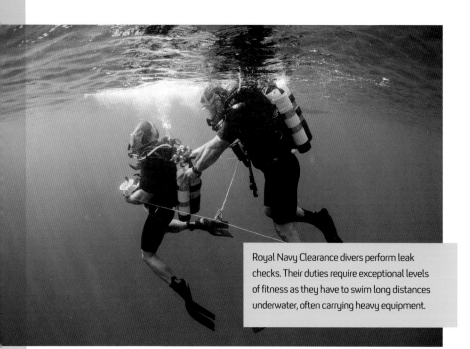

Royal Navy Clearance divers perform leak checks. Their duties require exceptional levels of fitness as they have to swim long distances underwater, often carrying heavy equipment.

Potential Diver Assessment (PDA)

This is a taster of the tests and exercises recruits are asked to perform under close professional supervision.

- 1,094yd (1,000m) swim across a lake in a dry suit, wearing flippers.
- Team challenge exercise. This can involve a 30-minute "Mud Crossing Techniques" exercise. The test is designed to reflect the reality divers sometimes face of carrying heavy equipment in an estuary.
- Trial dives in an enclosed tank in a lake. Recruits use a Swimmer Air Breathing Apparatus (SABA) to dive to a maximum depth of 23ft (7m).

This is followed by ten weeks' Initial Naval Training at HMS *Raleigh* in Torpoint, Devon, after which recruits go on an intensive phase two training course at DDS. This includes:

- Basic air diving
- Underwater maintenance and repair
- Underwater search operations
- Mixed gas diving
- Recompression operations
- Deep diving
- Diving equipment maintenance
- Bomb and mine disposal
- First aid
- Boat diving skills

Diver Personal Fitness Test (DPFT)

You can attempt some of these fitness tests, taking into account the usual common sense considerations for health and safety.

1. 1.5-mile (2.4km) run

This is equivalent to running six times round a standard athletic training track.
Aim: To test cardiorespiratory efficiency (stamina). This is to ensure that the potential diver will be physically robust enough to swim against tidal streams and river currents over an extended period.
Method: First you should do a warm-up run of 1.5 miles (2.4km) in 15 minutes (in the real test this will be conducted as a group). The next stage of the test is a 1.5-mile (2.4km) personal best effort.

Pass mark: The personal effort run must be completed in under 10:30 minutes.

2. Heaves (chin-ups)

Aim: The aim of this test is to assess shoulder (pull) strength. The reason this is so important is because a diver needs to be able to get out of the water unaided or may need to pull up equipment or an injured diver from the water.

Method:

- Grasp a secure fixed horizontal bar with arms fully extended, feet clear of the ground
- Place your hands in the under-grasp position
- Bend your arms and raise your body until the bottom of your chin is level with the top of the horizontal bar
- Lower yourself to full arm extension
- Repeat the exercise
- You are not allowed to swing on the bar during the test

Pass mark: At least eight heaves.

3. Flat and bent bench trunk curls

Aim: To measure your core strength/endurance. The test assesses your practical ability to lift objects from the water and also your overall fitness and stamina.

Method:

- On a flat bench, curl your trunk up and forward until your upper body is vertical
- Return in a controlled manner to the start position
- Your shoulderblades must touch the bench, while your feet should be secured at the upper end of the bench

- Your hands must touch the sides of your head at all times
- A bend at the knees is permitted

Pass mark: At least 40 trunk curls completed in 1 minute.

4. Dips

Aim: The aim of this test is to measure arm and shoulder (push) strength. From a practical point of view, this tests the ability of a diver to assist in the removal of injured divers or equipment from the water.

Method:

- Start with a straight-arm position on parallel bars or any two secure hand grips mounted above waist level and shoulder-width apart
- With your body supported in the vertical position and your feet clear of the ground, lower your body to achieve a right angle between the upper arm and forearm
- Return to the start position by straightening your arms
- Repeat the exercise

Pass mark: At least 16 dips.

5. Strength test

Aim: To measure your overall core body strength. From a practical point of view, to test the ability of a diver to carry heavy equipment from one place to another. One example of this could be to carry a full fuel container from a fuel stowage to a boat.

Method: You should lift two hand weights (66lb/30kg dumb bells or power bags) using the correct lifting technique and stand with one weight in each hand, maintaining an upright posture. You should then walk along a 33yd (30m) measured course. There is no time limit for this exercise.

Pass mark: You must complete the full 33yd (30m) course.

KAMPFSCHWIMMER

This is a German naval commando unit that is trained to operate by land, sea, and air. They are key special operations forces of the German Armed Forces, or Bundeswehr. Although about 70 percent of Kampfschwimmer operations are carried out on land, they often use water to approach their objectives unseen. Kampfschwimmer commandos are also trained in static-line, High Altitude High Opening (HAHO), and High Altitude Low Opening (HALO) parachute jumps, as well as fast-roping, rappeling, or Special Patrol Insertion/Extraction (SPIE) insertions.

The Basic Fitness Test

This test includes three elements:

Sprint test

11 × 33ft (10m) in under 60 seconds.

- Lie flat on your stomach on a mat, with your head pointing in the direction of movement and your hands folded on your back
- Jump up and sprint towards two markers, placed 33ft (10m) away
- Go round them and sprint back to the mat
- Resume the start prone position
- Spring up and repeat the sprint

After the fifth repetition there and back, sprint towards the markers. The test is ended when you pass them.

Hang test

Hang on a pull-up bar for a minimum of 5 seconds.

- Hold the pull-up bar with your thumb on the outside
- Place your hands shoulder-width apart
- Pull yourself up until your shoulders are level with the bar
- Hold for as long as possible

1,094yd (1,000m) track run

Completed in a maximum of 390 seconds.

11 x 33ft (10m) sprint test and hang test

Sprint Test		Hang Test		Rating
Seconds	Points	Seconds	Points	
60	99.98	5	100	100 points = passable
53.99	200.15	25	200	200 points = satisfactory
47.99	300.15	45	300	300 points = good
41.99	400.15	65	400	400 points = very good
35.99	500.15	85	500	500 points = excellent

Kampfschwimmer Entry

A series of stringent criteria must be met before the recruit can even be assessed for admission onto the basic diving course. If they pass, the recruit starts an eight-week dive training course.

Basic Diving Course entry test

- Run 3.1 miles (5km) within 25 minutes
- Swim 328yd (300m) fully clothed within 8 minutes
- Complete a minimum of three pull-ups
- Dive to a depth of 16ft (5m) and retrieve two 11lb (5kg) rings
- Swim 27yd (25m) underwater
- Qualify for the bronze life-saving badge, a complex test that involving various swimming, diving, and life-saving challenges

Kampfschwimmer Entrance Exam

After completion of the Basic Diving Course, recruits are eligible to take the Kampfschwimmer Entrance Exam.

- Run 3.1 miles (5km) within 22 minutes
- Swim 1,094yd (1,000m) within 24 minutes
- Submerge and hold your breath for a minimum of 60 seconds
- Swim 33yd (30m) underwater without surfacing (performing a half-turn halfway)
- Complete a minimum of eight pull-ups
- Benchpress a minimum of 110lb (50kg) for 15 repetitions

These are the minimum qualification standards. Recruits should aim to exceed them by a comfortable margin.

KUSTJÄGARNA

Sweden has an extensive coastline which during the Cold War was subject to probes by Soviet submarines and Spetznaz special forces. To some extent, this continues today. To monitor this threat, Sweden established the Kustjägarna (Coastal Rangers) special force in 1959. They are part of the Swedish Amphibious Corps, which in turn is part of the Swedish Navy. Modeled on special operations units such as the British Special Boat Service and US Navy SEALs, the Kustjägarna are trained for raids, coastal reconnaissance, and as a spearhead for larger force actions.

Coast Ranger Selection Course

To apply for the Kustjägarna, recruits must already be serving members of the Swedish Armed Forces. Recruits undergo the Coast Ranger Selection Course, which lasts for about two and a half days. Tests include the following:

- **Step-up test:** Carrying a 66lb (30kg) pack, you step up and down with the same leg for 3 minutes and then, after a brief rest, you do the same with the other foot for 3 minutes

- **Push-ups:** A minimum of 40 repetitions

- **Sit-ups:** A minimum of 40 repetitions

- **Static back hang:** Hang from a bar for at least 60 seconds

- **Military pull-up:** At least eight repetitions (hands palm forward on the bar)

- **Running:** 16 miles (10km) in under 49 minutes

- A swimming and water experience test, including breaststroke, lifesaving, and other water exercises

Coastal Ranger Basic Course

That is only the first hurdle. If they pass the selection, recruits move on to the Coastal Ranger Basic Course, where further tests include:

- A forced march over 3.2 miles (5.2km) with a 45lb (20kg) pack to be completed in under 42 minutes
- A fast march in hilly terrain over 4 miles (6.5km) with a 45lb (20kg) pack to be completed in under 40 minutes
- A four-day endurance exercise
- A distance kayak paddle of 120 nautical miles (138miles/222km)

The Kustjägarna are divided into Kustjägarna/KJ (commando unit) and Attackdykarna/A-DYK (frogmen). The commando has an assault priority while the frogmen are trained for reconnaissance. The Kustjägarna commandos operate from fast motor boats such as the Warboat 90, which is capable of traveling at 35 knots (40mph/65kph). It can come to a stop within 33ft (10m) from full speed. They are also trained for silent insertion by kayak and canoe. The divers have to undergo a 3.2-mile (2km) swim between two islands and reach their objective within 33ft (10m).

> # KUSTJÄGARNA COMMANDOS ARE TRAINED FOR SILENT INSERTION BY KAYAK

Part of the role of the Kustjagarna is to monitor and patrol the thousands of islands in the Swedish coastal archipelagos. This means that they have to be fit enough to endure very long kayak patrols over hundreds of miles and then be ready to carry out reconnaissance on land. They also have to be fit enough to endure the extreme cold of a northern winter.

On land, the Kustjagarna are skilled skiers, skiing long distances across country. They learn advanced cold weather survival skills, including building shelters in the snow, such as snow caves. They are trained to carry out operations from the cold weather bases and to survive in them for long periods.

DUTCH AMPHIBIOUS RECONNAISSANCE PLATOON

The Amfibisch Verkenningspeloton/Amphibious Reconnaissance Platoon (AMVERKPEL) is part of the Maritime Special Operations (MSO), one of three special forces under the Netherland Maritime Special Operations Force (NLMARSOF). Recruits must pass a variety of physical tests and also prove that they are up to it mentally.

Selection and Training

There is a 22-week selection and training course, with a failure rate of about 70 percent. The course includes:

- Naval diving
- Klepper canoe course
- Inland diving operations
- Reconnaissance, escape, and evasion techniques
- Counter-terrorist skills
- Endurance test

The joint special forces fitness test includes:

- 1.7-mile (2.8km) run in 12 minutes
- 40 push-ups in 2 minutes
- 60 sit-ups in 2 minutes
- 50 squats in 2 minutes
- 8 pull-ups in their own time
- EVO (basic vocational training) swimming test
- 10-mile (16km) run in 45 minutes
- 6.2-mile (10km) battle run with 33lb (15kg) of equipment, without water and within 60 minutes

> ## RECRUITS MUST PASS A VARIETY OF PHYSICAL TESTS AND PROVE THAT THEY ARE UP TO IT MENTALLY

The Elite of the Elite

The 7 NL SBS (Amfibish Veterennings Peloton) is a sub-unit of the Dutch Group of Operational Units Marines, including 1st Marine Battalion. Under the arrangements for the United Kingdom/Netherlands Amphibious Force (UKNLAF), the Dutch unit operates in conjunction with Britain's Marine 3 Commando Brigade in time of war. The unit is elite and small, limited to 25–26 men, subdivided into small teams. Responsibilities include long-range reconnaissance, small-scale raiding, training the Dutch navy in anti-mine and security procedures, and conducting anti-terrorist tasks.

Other units under the umbrella of the NLMARSOF include the Marine Intervention Unit (UIM) and the Maritime Special Operations Company (MSO). The MSO is divided into a mountain unit and a frogman unit. The mountain troops are specialized in both high altitude and extreme cold operations. The frogmen are specialized in amphibious reconnaissance.

NETHERLANDS MARINE CORPS

The Netherlands Marine Corps is part of the Royal Netherlands Navy. Like their counterparts in other national forces, Dutch marines are trained to carry out special maritime operations and amphibious landings while also being capable of operating effectively on land. To join the Netherlands Marine Corps, recruits need to pass the following tests:

- ☑ *1.6-mile (2.7km) run in 12 minutes*
- ☑ *30 push-ups in 2 minutes*
- ☑ *4 pull-ups in 2 minutes*

- ☑ *30 sit-ups in 2 minutes*
- ☑ *A strength endurance test*

BRITISH ROYAL MARINES

The Royal Marines are an elite commando unit of the Royal Navy. They are kept in a high state of readiness in order to respond quickly to emergencies around the world. The Marines are trained to be highly mobile and independent and to carry out high impact operations, from seaborne assaults on land, to mountainous cold weather operations. You don't get much tougher than this, so if you can match any of the Royal Marines tests, you are doing very well.

Royal Marines Pre-Joining Fitness Test

Before a recruit goes anywhere near the Royal Marines they need to pass the Royal Marines Pre-Joining Fitness Test, which involves two runs on a treadmill set at a 2 percent incline. The first run should be completed in under 12:30 minutes and the second run immediately afterwards in less than 10 minutes.

Royal Marines Basic Fitness Test

Royal Marines minimum entry requirements in the Royal Marines Basic Fitness Test (RMBFT) include:

- Five pull-ups in your own time
- 50 sit-ups in under 2 minutes

- A squad run and walk of 1.5 miles (2.4km) in under 15 minutes
- A best-effort run of 1.5 miles (2.4km) in under 11:30 minutes

Those who attend the All Arms Commando Course (AACC) or Royal Marines Young Officers' Course (RMYOC) will also need to accomplish the following on top of the RMBFT:

- Swim 66yd (60m) in clothing and tread water for 3 minutes
- Be capable of traversing a standard military assault course in boots
- Be able to perform the Fireman's Carry with the correct technique (the recruit

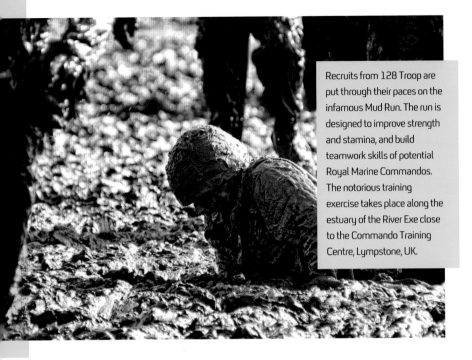

Recruits from 128 Troop are put through their paces on the infamous Mud Run. The run is designed to improve strength and stamina, and build teamwork skills of potential Royal Marine Commandos. The notorious training exercise takes place along the estuary of the River Exe close to the Commando Training Centre, Lympstone, UK.

carries the other person across their shoulders with one arm and one leg in front of their body, with the recruit's arm tucked round the leg and holding the arm, see photograph, page 135)

■ Be able to climb a minimum of 30ft (9m) of rope in boots and denims using a good technique (see page 164)

Royal Marines Commando Test

These tests take place at Commando Training Centre Royal Marines (CTCRM) and comprise the following:

■ **Endurance course:** Wearing full combat equipment and carrying a weapon, recruits must pass through 2 miles (3.2km) of tunnels and woods before running 4 miles (6.4km) back to camp. The course should be completed in under 72 minutes. Back at camp, they have to score 6 out of 10 in a shooting test.

■ **Speed march:** Recruits must complete 9 miles (14.5km) in under 90 minutes, carrying equipment and a rifle.

■ **Tarzan assault course:** This includes rope climbs, a zip line, and a 30ft (9m) wall. The course should be completed in 13 minutes.

■ **30-mile (48km) march:** Needs to be completed within 8 hours/7 hours for officers.

US MARINE CORPS

The United States Marine Corps is an elite force that is capable of fighting from land, sea, and air simultaneously. The US Marines operate as highly mobile expeditionary units. US Marines are trained to fight in all terrains and temperature zones from arctic and mountain through desert to jungle. They have a global reach.

The Marine Corps includes a number of specialist sub-units, including the 1st Reconnaissance Battalion 1st Marine Division (often known as Marine Recon). The Marines also have a unique scout sniper unit, which combines reconnaissance and sniper roles. The Marines also have their own special forces under US Marine Corps Special Operations Command (MARSOC). The US Marine Corps Initial Strength Test (IST) for recruits is a shortened version of the US Marine Corps Physical Fitness Test that every Marine undertakes every six months. The IST is fairly straightforward, involving only push-ups,

sit-ups, and a 1.5 mile (2.4km) run but the Marine Corps emphasize that this is the absolute minimum standard. In order to have a successful career as a Marine the recruit will be expected to perform comfortably above that.

US Marine Corps Combat Fitness Test (CFT)

This 300-point test is designed to reflect real operational demands. Every Marine has to take the test once a year, though there are different scoring criteria for males and females as well as age groups. The test consists of the following three parts:

Movement to contact

This is a 880yd (805m) sprint that is performed outside as fast as possible. Maximum score is 2:45 minutes for males or 3:23 minutes for females.

Ammunition lift

Marines must lift a 30lb (14kg) ammunition can over their heads until their arms lock as many times as possible. (If you want to try this test, a large carton of water of the same weight may be a substitute.) The can is lifted until the elbows lock, and is then lowered until it is below chin level. The time limit is 2 minutes in which to complete as many repetitions as possible. The maximum score for males is 91 lifts. The maximum score for females is 61 lifts.

Maneuver under fire

This demanding part of the test most closely reflects real combat conditions. The recruit must sprint to a 25yd (23m) line and perform a hook turn round the marker before taking up a high-crawl position and high crawling for 10yd (9m). At the 35yd (32m) line they must perform a modified high crawl for 15yd (14m) to the 50yd (46m) line. They then sprint through the markers to the 75yd (69m) line. At the 75yd line a simulated casualty (or sandbag) is dragged 10yd

(9m) through the first two cones at the 65yd (59m) line. Once past the second cone the simulated casualty is lifted into the Fireman's Carry position. The simulated casualty is carried 65yd (59m) straight back to the starting line. Two 30lb (14kg) ammunition cans (you could use water jerricans) must then be carried back to the 75yd (69m) line. A dummy grenade (or a large stone) is then thrown at the grenade target from a standing position.

The recruit performs three push-ups, and ammunition cans (or water jerricans) are carried back to the start line. The goal is to complete the course as fast as possible.

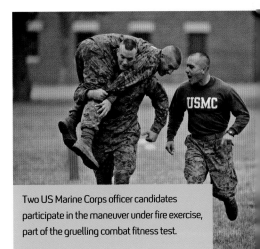

Two US Marine Corps officer candidates participate in the maneuver under fire exercise, part of the gruelling combat fitness test.

US NAVY SEALS

The US Navy SEALs today are trained to the highest standards and are ready to move at any time to engage in direct action (to neutralize enemy forces), or to conduct special reconnaissance (to observe and report), or counter-terrorism (to eliminate threats). To become a Navy SEAL, recruits have to meet high physical and mental standards before they even start training. Special forces have to perform in some of the most challenging environments in the world and in situations which require not only extreme physical fitness but also quick-thinking. Endurance and stamina have to be both mental and physical.

Preliminary Requirements

To join the US Navy SEALs, recruits need to be a member of the US Navy, which means that they have already met certain standards of fitness and mental ability. They will be subjected to various screening tests to assess their abilities, including pre-enlistment medical screening, the Armed Services Vocational Aptitude Battery (ASVAB), the Armed Forces Qualification Test (AFQT), the Computerized Special Operations Resilience Test (C-SORT), and the SEAL Physical Screening Test (PST).

Physical Screening Test

The physical screening test for budding SEALs is divided into minimum and optimum scores. Navy SEALs need to be physically fit as well as resilient and tenacious. Training for SEALs will include activities such as running in soft sand for long periods carrying heavy equipment. They also need to be at home in the water and able to swim long distances, both on the surface and underwater. Swimming may need to be performed fully clothed. In real operations, Navy SEALs often emerge from the ocean or rivers fully clothed, carrying a weapon and ready for action.

Physical screening test

Test	Minimum	Optimum
Swim 500yd (457m)	12:30 min	9:00 min
Push-ups	50	90
Curl-ups	50	85
Pull-ups	10	18
Run 1.5 miles (2.4km)	10:30 min	9:30 min

Swim test

The strokes required for the tests are either breaststroke or sidestroke. Both strokes are to be performed without overhand recovery; in other words, the swimmer's hands must remain below the surface at all times. After entering the water, swimmers may push off from the sides with their hands and feet after each length. Swimmers can rest by using the survival float or by treading water.

Push-ups

In the "up" position, arms should be straight and back, buttocks, and legs should be in line. In the "down" position, the arms form a right angle and the back, buttocks, and legs are in line. The upper arms should be parallel to the deck. The candidate can only rest in the "up" position.

Curl-ups

In the test, the feet are held by a companion. Hands must remain in contact with the shoulders or chest at all times. Elbows should touch the knees or no more than 3in (8cm) below the knees. The recruit lies flat on the ground with their knees bent and their heels no more than 10in (25cm) from their buttocks. The timer calls out 15-second time intervals until 2 minutes have elapsed.

Pull-ups

The recruit starts in the dead-hang position, with arms and shoulders fully extended. Their palms should be shoulder-width apart and they should have an overhand grip on the bar. The recruit pulls their body up until their chin is level with or over the bar. They can cross their legs but must not jerk or swing the body. They then lower the body again until the arms are fully extended.

1.5-mile (2.4km) run

The run is performed in running shirt, shorts, and trainers. A timer calls out the laps each time the recruit passes. The run is to be completed as fast as possible.

US AIR FORCE SPECIAL OPERATIONS COMMAND

US Air Force Special Operations Command (AFSOC) is part of US Special Operations Command (USSOCOM). Their objective is to provide special operations airmen for a variety of missions on a global basis. Special operations roles include combat rescue officers, combat controllers, pararescue, weather teams, and tactical air controllers.

Physical Fitness Entry Requirements

Here the fitness entry requirements reflect the range of capabilities that are required of special forces personnel:

- 2 × 22yd (20m) underwater with 3 minutes between each (followed by a 10-minute rest)
- 547yd (500m) swim (this can be freestyle, breaststroke, or sidestroke) in under 14 minutes (followed by a 30-minute rest)
- A 1.5-mile (2.4km) run in 10 minutes and 45 seconds (followed by a 10-minute rest)
- Pull-ups in under 1 minute with minimum 6 repetitions (followed by a 3-minute rest)
- Push-ups in under 2 minutes, with minimum 45 repetitions (followed by a 3-minute rest)
- Flutter kicks in under 2 minutes, with minimum 45 repetitions

AFSOC Specialist Roles

The AFSOC includes a number of specialist roles:

Combat Controller

The USAF Combat Controller course is one of the toughest courses in the US Air

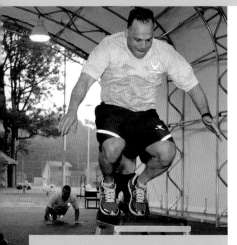

US airmen perform circuit training, which is excellent preparation for the range of tasks and obstacles that they are likely to be presented with on a battlefield.

Force. Combat Controllers often work on attachment to other special forces units and they have the responsibility of coordinating close air support (CAS) while maneuvering with the unit. While being capable of accompanying any special forces unit to their objective by air, land, or sea, these specialized airmen have all the skills of a fully fledged Air Traffic Controller. Their involvement can make the difference between success or failure of a mission.

Combat Rescue Officer

Their mission is to recover injured personnel from the battlefield, which often means putting themselves in danger. In order to carry out their role, the CROs need to be extremely fit and to be able to infiltrate the area by air, overland, by static-line or freefall parachute, or by underwater diving.

Pararescue

These airmen work with Combat Rescue Officers to provide emergency medical treatment on and recovery from a battlefield or other emergency situation. This means that they have to be exceptionally fit and able to access the area by static-line or freefall parachuting or underwater diving. They must be able to operate in mountains, deserts, and a wide variety of other environments.

FORSVARETS SPESIALKOMMANDO

The Forsvarets Spesialkommando (FSK) is the Norwegian Special Operations command and it includes three major sub-units: Fallskjermjeger, Jegertroppen, and Spesialjeger. The special operations command was created to defend Norwegian interests both offshore (including oil and gas installations) and on land, and on operations abroad, such as Allied operations in Afghanistan. Recruits need to be serving members of the Norwegian Armed Forces.

Fallskjermjeger (Paratroopers)

To join the Norwegian paratroop corps you need to be a conscript in the Norwegian armed forces. The elite paratroop corps operate in six-man teams that carry out both reconnaissance and offensive operations after insertion by air, using either High Altitude High Opening (HAHO), High Altitude Low Opening (HALO), or static jumps.

Jegertroppen (Rangers)

This ranger unit is made up of female conscripts. The Jegertroppen rangers are primarily tasked with working in small units on reconnaissance missions. This demands a high level of physical fitness, specialist skills (e.g. communications and navigation), and the ability to work both independently and in small teams. Those that pass boot camp will go on to specialist training in parachuting, handgun shooting, driving skills, survival, and information retrieval.

Spesialjeger (Special Forces)

Norwegian special forces operators have a wide remit that includes reconnaissance, surveillance, offensive operations, and counter-terrorism. The selection process for special forces takes two years. Training includes weapons and shooting skills, insertion by parachute, driving, communications, and medical and survival training.

Recruits for Forsvarets Spesialkommando (Armed Forces Special Command) need to pass a number of fitness tests, including the minimum entrance test and the more advanced special operations test. As with all special operations entrance tests, they need to do much better than minimum standard if they want to get ahead. See if you can match the standard.

> JEGERTROPPEN RANGERS NEED A HIGH LEVEL OF FITNESS AND SPECIALIST SKILLS

Minimum requirements

- 5 pull-ups
- 30 push-ups
- 35 sit-ups in 2 minutes
- 20 deadlifts
- Swimming 219yd (200m) in 6 minutes. You may have a diving start. Underwater swim without goggles.
- 4.3-mile (7km) road race with a 33lb (15kg) pack to be completed in 49 minutes. This test is conducted on country roads.

Candidates who make it through to recruit school are tested again on their fitness, with the standards raised all round. The tests are designed to measure the physical improvement that should have taken place during the duration of boot camp. They are as follows:

- 6 pull-ups
- 35 push-ups
- 45 sit-ups in under 2 minutes
- 20 deadlifts
- 4.3-mile (7km) speed march with a 49lb (22kg) pack and a weapon, wearing full combat kit. The march should be completed in under 50 minutes.

PARACHUTE RECONNAISSANCE COMPANY 17

This is a specialized unit of the Swiss KSK. The unit is responsible for reconnaissance missions that require paratroop drops as well as long-range patrols. Members of the unit are trained in High Altitude Low Opening (HALO) and High Altitude High Opening (HAHO) parachute drops onto both land and water.

Entry Test

The entry test is made up of push-ups, sit-ups, and a 12-minute run, with very specific parameters.

Push-ups

The Swiss physical entry test push-ups are different from the standard push-ups found in many other physical fitness tests. The following sequence must be completed within 2 minutes:

- Lie face down on a mat, with your hands behind your back
- Push yourself up with your hands so that your back is straight and you are supported on your hands and toes
- Touch your right hand with your left hand while supporting yourself with your right arm
- Lower yourself onto your chest and touch your two hands together across your back
- Raise yourself again and once again touch your right hand with your left
- Lower yourself and touch your hands across your back
- Raise yourself and touch your left hand with your right hand, while supporting yourself with your left arm

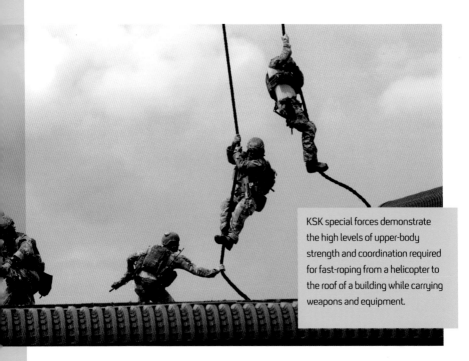

KSK special forces demonstrate the high levels of upper-body strength and coordination required for fast-roping from a helicopter to the roof of a building while carrying weapons and equipment.

Sit-ups

You get one point for every repetition in this part of the test.

- Lie on your back on a mat, with your body and legs straight and your arms stretched on the ground above your head
- Raise your torso using your abdominal muscles and simultaneously bring your knees up toward your chest
- Clutch your arms briefly around your ankles
- Lower yourself to the previous flat position
- Repeat

12-minute run

You must run at maximum pace and the distance you have run on the track will be recorded. If you run between 1.5 and 1.7 miles (2.4 and 2.7km) in the time you will be considered above average. Any faster than that and maybe you should consider the Olympics...

TEST METHODS, SKILLS, AND STRATEGIES

It's not what you do but the way that you do it that really counts. Nothing could be more true of military tests. First, you won't pass the test unless you've got the technique right (yes, those arms have to be at 90 degrees in the push-up…) and, second, getting the technique right from the start will make your training and preparation more efficient and reduce the risk of injury. For example, it will make the difference between success and failure if you get your arm movements right when doing a standing long-jump, while if you have been practicing pull-ups with an underhand grip when the test demands an overhand grip, you will have wasted your time.

It is also useful to know exactly which muscles are being used in each test so that you can reflect on the optimum training, stretching, warm-ups, and cool-downs for those specific muscle groups.

Practice makes perfect. Once you have refined your technique, you can then focus on practicing with the confidence that you are training the right muscles in the right way. Preparation is the key to success, said Alexander Graham Bell. By reading this chapter and following the advice, you will be well on the way to achieving your goal.

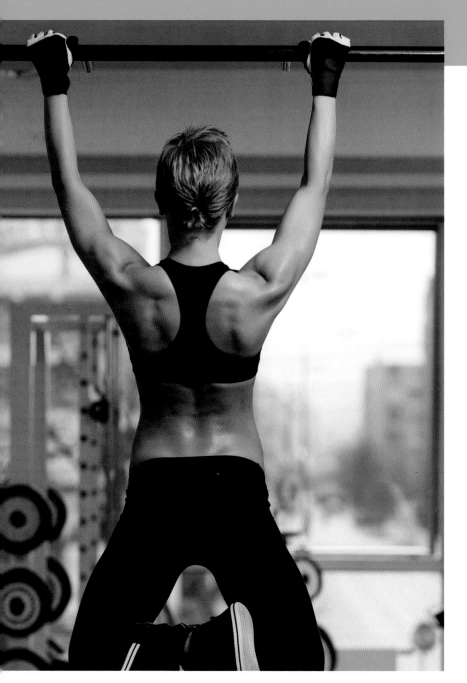

PULL-UPS

Many fitness experts consider pull-ups to be among the best tests of upper-body strength, and many armed forces use them both for testing and for improving and maintaining upper-body strength and endurance. The tests are often not timed, the recruit being allowed to continue as long as he or she is able.

Variants

There are many styles of pull-up. Variables include hand width, hand grip (over- or underhand), leg position (straight, bent, or crossed), height of the pull required (e.g., chin above the bar, chest to the bar), whether the elbows must be locked straight at the bottom of each repetition ("dead hang"), orientation to the bar (e.g., sideways), one-handed, weighted, and others. Some consider a true pull-up to be one in which an overhand—or pronated—grip is used (with the palms facing forward), and a chin-up to be one with an underhand or supinated grip (with the palms facing back). This terminology is not accepted consistently, however, and various militaries use the terms indiscriminately while requiring one grip or the other or even permitting a choice. Tests also vary in the amount of lower body movement permitted, from none to almost unlimited.

Strategies

Pull-up test performance can be enhanced by adopting the following strategies, if allowed:

- Use the pronated grip (palms facing away from you).
- Place hands shoulder-width apart or wider on the bar.
- Cross your ankles and draw your legs up as much as possible, bending at the hips and the knees to minimize swinging.

PULL-UPS

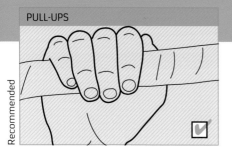

PULL-UPS

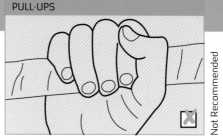

CHIN-UPS

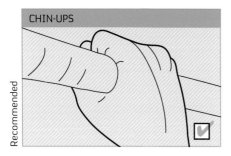

CHIN-UPS

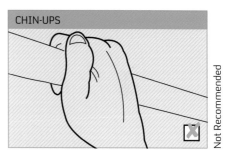

- On the other hand, if unlimited lower body movement is allowed, "kipping" helps a great deal. This involves vigorously swinging your body to create upward momentum before you begin to pull with your arms.

- Begin by ripping off as many reps as you can, as quickly as possible, then pause at a dead hang for a few seconds to regain your strength before making a final effort for a few last ups.

Training Tips

Pull-ups are one of the rare test events for which the best training may be the same exercise. If you can do no pull-ups at all, start with "negatives." Use a stool or have a friend boost you to the up position, with your chin above the bar. Hold yourself there for 5 seconds, then slowly lower yourself down to a dead hang and hold yourself for another 5 seconds before repeating the cycle.

MUSCLES WORKED

- ☑ Latissimus dorsi (back)
- ☑ Brachialis (upper arm)
- ☑ Brachioradialis (forearm)
- ☑ Biceps (upper arm)
- ☑ Triceps (upper arm)

- ☑ Teres major (upper arm)
- ☑ Rhomboids (upper back)
- ☑ Trapezius (upper back and neck)
- ☑ Levator scalpulae (back/side of neck)

- ☑ Deltoid (shoulder)
- ☑ Abdominal muscles
- ☑ Pelvic muscles
- ☑ Hands

PUSH-UPS

The push-up, or press-up, is one of the most common forms of fitness training and testing. Without the use of external weights, this exercise uses the body's own weight to test upper-body strength, especially in the arms, shoulders, and chest, but also in the abdomen, hips, and legs. It also demands a high degree of proprioception, namely the body's ability to maintain a regular position in order to carry out the proper technique. As it is so common, the push-up can all too easily be done with the wrong technique. In testing, if the technique is wrong, the push-up will not be counted.

Variants

Wide push-up: Place your hands 6in (15cm) wider than your shoulders on both sides and then perform the push-up in the usual way.

Triceps push-up: Place your hands pointing inwards in order to focus the strain on your triceps muscles.

Knee push-up: This is a push-up with your knees resting on the ground.

Bench push-up: This can either be done by placing your feet on a secure bench and doing the push-up in the usual way or by placing your hands on a bench and pushing up.

Wall push-up: This can be a good exercise when you are a beginner and you are still getting used to the push-up technique. You can start by leaning against a wall and then carrying out the push-up motion against the wall. Then move your feet a little further from the wall in order to increase the pressure on your arms and until you feel ready to do the full horizontal push-up.

Strategies

In order to perform a correct military push-up, follow these guidelines:

- Get on the ground with your hands on the floor, shoulder-width apart, with

WIDE PUSH-UP

KNEE PUSH-UP

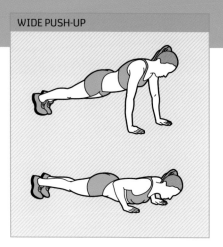

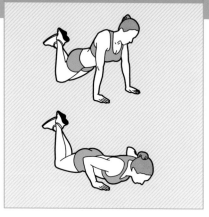

your fingers pointing forward. Your legs should be straight and you should be resting on your toes. Your feet can either be together or shoulder-width apart.

- Keep your back straight. Your neck should also be straight. Look either forward or downward.
- Concentrate on your core muscles to keep your body rigid.
- Keeping your body straight, bend your arms to a roughly 90-degree angle from shoulder to elbow and lower yourself until your chest is about ¾–1⅛in (2–3cm) from the floor. Keep your arms close to your chest at all times.

- Push up again until your arms lock. Some service tests allow women to perform the push-up with their knees on the ground. Otherwise, their arms and body position should be the same as for the full traditional push-up.

Training Tips

Some military entrance tests, particularly for elite and special forces, require you to perform at least 50 push-ups. This will require a lot of training. Normally a day's rest should be allowed to allow muscle to rebuild, but some fitness gurus argue that push-ups can be done every day, in sets of, say, ten, to achieve a maximum of 100 a day, building up to 200 a day.

MUSCLES WORKED

- ☑ Pectorals (chest)
- ☑ Triceps (back of upper arm)

- ☑ Deltoids (shoulder)
- ☑ Serratus anterior (upper ribs)

- ☑ Coracobrachialis (upper and medial arm)

SIT-UPS

Along with push-ups, sit-ups are one of the standard fitness test exercises in military assessments. The main muscle groups tested by the sit-up are core abdominal strength, as well as the back and legs. The sit-up is an important exercise for maintaining a stable body core, which acts as a firm base for a wide range of exercises and activities. It also helps proof the body against injuries, such as lower back injury. A typical minimum standard for sit-ups is 50, though some military tests ask for the maximum number until exhaustion.

Variants

There are two broad divisions between sit-ups: the supported and unsupported. With the supported sit-up, the feet are held down by a companion or tucked under a stable object. The supported sit-up places more strain on the lower back and should not be used if you have a lower back weakness or injury.

Supported sit-up 1

- Lie on your back. Keeping your feet flat, move them toward your body so that your legs are bent at 90 degrees.
- Keep your arms straight. Place your palms on top of your upper legs.

- Tuck your chin toward your chest and sit up, sliding your hands along your upper thighs and past the knees. Stop once your wrists pass your knee caps.
- Lower yourself slowly to the start position within about 3 seconds.

Supported sit-up 2

- Lie on your back and, keeping your feet flat on the floor, bring them in to create a 90-degree angle.
- Place your hands behind or next to your head, with your elbows back. Gently cradle your head with your hands—do not pull on your head as this may cause a neck injury.

SUPPORTED SIT-UP

UNSUPPORTED SIT-UP

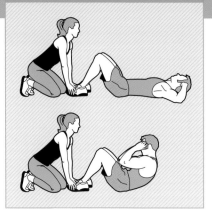

- Slowly curl your body toward your knees, keeping your neck straight and looking straight ahead at all times.
- Then slowly lower yourself back down to the start position.

Unsupported sit-up 1
- Lie flat on the ground with your arms stretched behind your head.
- Sit up, keeping your arms straight, until your chest meets your knees, with your arms pointing straight ahead over your knees.
- Then lower yourself down, placing your arms flat on the ground as before.

Unsupported sit-up 2
To vary your training, you can try an unsupported sit up with your legs remaining straight on the ground and your arms pointing forward, horizontal with the ground.

Strategies
While performing sit-ups, keep your breathing regular. It is best to inhale as you lower your body so that you do not have to push against your full lungs as you raise your body. Tense your abdominal muscles before you attempt to rise up. Make sure that you keep your lower back on the ground. Do not pull up with your neck.

MUSCLES WORKED

- ☑ *Rectus abdominis (vertical abdominal muscle)*
- ☑ *Obliquus externus abdominis (external abdominals)*

- ☑ *Tensor fasciae latae (thigh)*
- ☑ *Rectus femoris (quad muscle in upper leg)*
- ☑ *Iliopsoas (hip)*
- ☑ *Sartorius (thigh)*

DIPS

Tricep dips have often been used in military testing. The dip uses the body weight and works both the elbow and shoulder joint. The dip is a popular military exercise because it adds greatly to overall upper-body strength and also improves balance, due to the fact that the upper-body muscles have to work hard to stabilize the body as you lower and raise yourself.

Variants

Dips can be done either with a bench or between parallel bars. If using a bench, make sure it is sturdy and secure. Bend your legs and place your palms on the front edge of the bench, with fingers pointing forward. Push your feet out in front of you so that your body weight is mostly resting on your arms. Then slowly bend your arms and lower your body until your upper arms are parallel to the floor. Do not go lower from this point. Start to raise your body again to the previous position to complete one dip. If using parallel bars, grasp the bars firmly with your hands, tuck your feet up so that you are off the ground and lower yourself until your upper arms are at 90 degrees to the ground before raising yourself up again.

Strategies

It is important to perform the exercise with slow rhythmic movements. When you are lowering yourself, make sure that your shoulders remain low and do not rise toward your ears. If you keep your hips close to the bench, it will maximize the strengthening of the triceps as opposed to the shoulder muscles. As you start your triceps training, keep your feet close in to the

DIP WITH BENCH

DIP WITH PARALLEL BARS

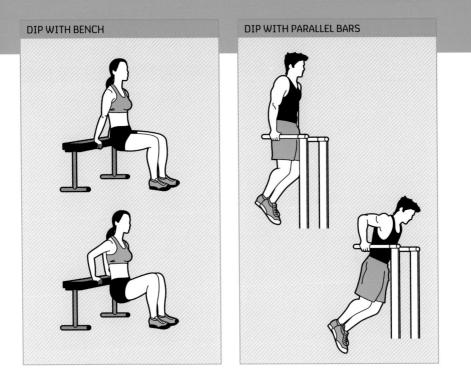

bench. As you get stronger, move your feet out gradually to increase the weight on your triceps.

Training Tips

Make sure you are looking forward when you do a dip, so as to keep your upper spine level. Take a deep breath before the dip and when you rise back up from the dip, as your muscle contractions will make it difficult to breathe. Try bending your legs and crossing your feet. Do some pull-ups as a complementary exercise.

MUSCLES WORKED

☑ Pectoralis major (chest muscle)
☑ Triceps brachii (back of upper arm)

LEG LIFTS

Leg lifts are an excellent way to strengthen the abdominal muscles, which in turn provide better support for the lower back. When performing a leg lift, the body has to perform more complex functions than may be immediately apparent. There is an isometric contraction involving abdominal muscles and hip flexors. The abdominals are involved not only in the lifting process, but also in keeping your torso stable.

Variants

Standard leg lift: This involves lifting both legs from a lying down position. Lie flat on the floor, looking straight upward so that your neck is relatively straight. Keeping your legs straight, lift your legs slowly off the ground until your heels are about 6in (15cm) from the ground. This is the start position. Now raise your legs further upward and then down to the start position. Repeat as many times as you can.

Single leg lift: This begins from the same start position. One leg is kept straight, and the other is lifted to an angle of 60 degrees, then back to the start position, before doing the same with the other leg.

Vertical leg lift: Lie on your back and raise both your legs so that they are vertical. You can cross your ankles to stabilize your legs. Keep your hands by your sides. Then lower your legs until your heels almost touch the ground before raising your legs back up again to the vertical position. You can also lift your head off the ground, taking care not to strain your neck, and move your hands further down beside your buttocks. Make sure the movements are slow and that there is no pressure on your back or

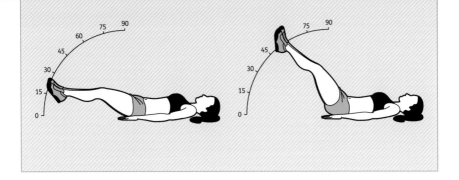

MUSCLES WORKED

- ☑ *Iliacus, pertineus, abductor longus (hip flexors)*
- ☑ *Transverse abdominis (abdominal)*
- ☑ *Obliques (abdominal)*

on your neck. Slow movements ensure that your abdominal muscles get the full benefit of the contractions that are involved in the exercise.

Bent leg lift: Lie on your back with your knees bent at 45 degrees and your feet flat on the ground. Then raise your legs until your thighs are perpendicular to the ground.

Strategies

Keep your back flat on the floor throughout the exercise and concentrate on contracting your abdominal muscles. When lying on your back, try to keep your stomach as tight as possible. Imagine pulling your navel down towards your back. This will also help focus the exercise on the transverse abdominis.

Training Tips

It is a good idea to warm up before you start leg lifts. This can be done by either a 5–10-minute walk or some light rowing (if you have a rowing machine). Try one or two sets of 10–12 lifts and move onto three sets when you are stronger.

SQUATS

When done properly, squats can help strengthen not only your leg muscles but your core as well. Squats are a popular choice in military tests as squatting down to pick up objects or even to take cover is an everyday military activity. Practicing squats helps your body to form the muscle groups that help you to maintain your balance as well as improving your strength. They also improve proprioception, the coordination between brain and muscle that helps you to perform activities efficiently.

Variants

Standard squat: Stand with feet shoulder-width apart and stretch your arms straight out in front of you. Turn your feet out slightly. Then slowly squat downward until your thighs are parallel to the floor. Push yourself back up again and repeat the exercise. An alternative method is to hold your arms straight up above your head (British Army requirement).

Split squat: Stand with feet shoulder-width apart. Step forward with one foot and back with the other. Your back foot should be on its toes. Fold your arms across your chest and, keeping your back straight, lower your hips straight down, placing the weight on the heel of your front foot. Keep lowering until your front knee is bent to 45 degrees. Push back up from your heel into the starting position. As you become more practiced and stronger, you will be able to take the split squat lower until your front leg is at 90 degrees.

Strategies

Keep your knees pointing forward when you squat. When you start training, keep your feet fairly wide to improve stability if necessary but bring them in as you get

STANDARD SQUAT

PISTOL SQUAT

MUSCLES WORKED

- ☑ *Semimembranosus (hamstrings)*
- ☑ *Gluteus maximus (buttocks)*
- ☑ *Semimembranosus (hip muscles)*

stronger so that your muscles are trained for stability. Keep your spine in a neutral position throughout.

Training Tips

To begin with, perform two or three sets of squats two or three times per week. It is important to allow your body some recovery time, so don't overdo it. As you get stronger, you should be able to perform more sets.

Although practicing standard squats is excellent and will probably help you to reach your target, variety is the spice of life and may also help to train your muscles more efficiently. Add some weights, which will make the straight body squat feel a lot easier when it comes to the test. Try the pistol squat, where you raise one leg off the floor in front of you and sink down on the other leg. The barbell squat involves holding a barbell across your shoulders when performing the squat. The weight squat involves holding a weight in your outstretched arms.

LUNGES

Lunges have a similar effect on the lower body to squats. They have the added benefit of demanding balance and coordination. Lunges exercise the quadriceps, or thigh muscles, the gluteus maximus, or buttocks, as well as the hamstrings. There are variations on lunges. They can be performed as part of your pre-exercise warm-up.

Variants

Standard lunge: Stand with your feet together and arms by your sides. Step forward with one leg and back with the other, resting your back foot on your toes. Fold your arms across your chest. Keep your back straight and lower your hips straight downward, placing the weight on the heel of your front foot, then lower your hips until your front knee is bent to 45 degrees. Push back up from your heel into the start position to complete the lunge.

Walking lunge: Keep moving forward, making the lunge on alternate legs.

Weighted lunge: Hold weights (e.g., 6.6lb/3kg) in your hands as you lunge.
Barbell lunge: Hold a barbell of a manageable weight securely across the back of your neck as you make the lunge.

Strategies

Keep breathing regularly when performing lunges in order to maximize effectiveness. As you lunge forward, exhale, and then inhale when you push yourself back into the start position. Make sure that your spine is straight throughout the movement and keep your shoulders over your hips. Before you start, flex your abdominal muscles both

STANDARD LUNGE

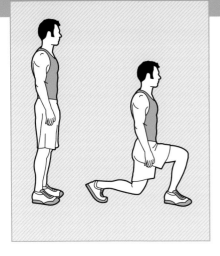

Training Tips

Try performing your lunges next to a mirror so that you can check for correct alignment. To gain maximum benefit from your lunge exercises, keep going until your heart rate has raised and your legs are too tired to continue.

inward and upward. Make sure you are standing straight before you start the lunge. Let your shoulders relax. The heel of the foot you are stepping forward with should be slightly lifted, so that you touch the ground with your forefoot. Try holding the lunge position for up to 5 seconds before starting to rise. To rise up from the lunge, place the pressure on the heel of your forward foot.

MUSCLES WORKED

- ☑ *Quadriceps (thigh)*
- ☑ *Gluteal muscles (buttocks)*
- ☑ *Semimembranosus (hamstrings)*
- ☑ *Adductor brevis, adductor longus, adductor magnus, pectineus, and gracilis (hip adductors)*
- ☑ *Gluteus minimus, gluteus maximus, gluteus medius, tensor fascia lata (hip adductors)*

STANDING LONG JUMP

The standing long jump, which is less usual in general sport than the running long jump, is used in military tests to assess your leg power as well as coordination. It has practical implications for jumping over or across obstacles in the course of military duties.

Variants

To perform the standing long jump, stand at the end of a long-jump landing mat with your feet slightly apart. Bend your knees, lean forward and jump in a forward and upward direction. When you land, bend your legs at the knees. Before you jump, your feet must be parallel and should not be touching the mat. The jump will be measured from the start of the mat to the closest indicator of where you landed (which is why you should not allow yourself to fall backward when you land). You are allowed three attempts and the best jump will be the one recorded.

Strategies

When preparing to jump, bend at the knees and hips to an angle of 90 degrees, as this will increase the power of your jump. Lean forward, so that when you push with your legs you are pushing both forward and upward. Swing both arms first backward straight out behind you and then, as you push up and forward with your legs, windmill your arms forward to add to the forward momentum. They should reach shoulder level just as your feet leave the ground. During the jump your feet should move forward while your arms move back toward your hips. As you land, you

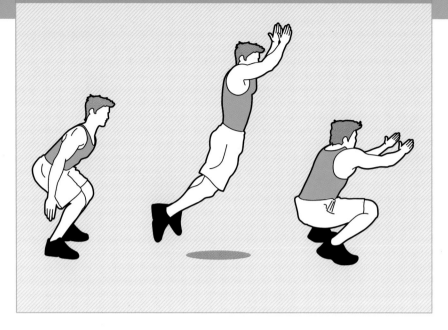

MUSCLES WORKED

☑ *Quadriceps femoris (thigh)*
☑ *Vastus medialis (thigh)*
☑ *Vastus intermedius (thigh)*
☑ *Vastus lateralis (thigh)*
☑ *Rectus femoris (thigh)*
☑ *Gluteus maximus (buttocks)*
☑ *Semimembranosus (hamstring)*

Training Tips

To practice the jump, use a sandpit or a mat for a soft landing and to avoid injury. Take a 2–3-minute break between jumps so that your body is fully recovered before the next jump. Squats are an excellent exercise to practice for standing jumps as they will build up your leg muscles and strengthen your back.

should try to extend your legs as far forward as possible. As your arms will also be forward, this helps you to keep your balance and will stop you from falling backward as you land.

VERTICAL JUMP

The vertical jump is not a regular feature in military fitness tests but it is used by some armed forces, including Spain and Sweden, to test leg power.

Variants

The vertical jump is usually performed against a wall with height markings on it. Stand side-on to a wall and reach up as high as you can with your arm closest to the wall. The point you reach will be marked as the standing reach height. Move a little away from the wall and jump up as high as possible. Either touch the measured scale on the wall with chalked hands or have the jump measured on the tape. Both feet must hit the ground simultaneously on landing. You are normally allowed three attempts and the best is recorded as your highest jump. Other forms of measurement include technical equipment such as a timing mat or jump mat.

With the pure squat jump, or static jump, you start from a stationary semi-squat position and cannot use your arms or any form of counter-movement.

Running vertical jump: With this variant you get the impetus of a run to power your jump. This mirrors the actions of a basketball player. It can be a good way of bringing some variety into your vertical jump training.

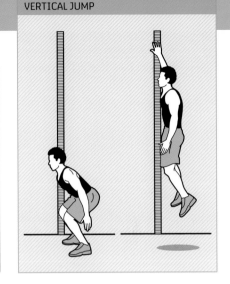

MUSCLES WORKED

- ☑ *Gluteus maximus (buttocks)*
- ☑ *Semitendinosus (hip to thigh)*
- ☑ *Semimembranosus (hamstring)*
- ☑ *Biceps femoris (back upper leg)*
- ☑ *Adductor magnus (thigh)*
- ☑ *Quadriceps femoris (thigh)*
- ☑ *Gastrocnemius (calf)*
- ☑ *Soleus (calf/ankle)*
- ☑ *Deltoid (shoulder)*
- ☑ *Supraspinatus (shoulder)*
- ☑ *Pectoralis major (chest)*

Strategies

When preparing to perform a vertical jump, stand in bare feet or socks on a mat. Keeping your back straight, place your hands on your hips and squat down until your knees are bent at 90 degrees. In military rules for the test, bending of the knees and trunk is allowed to perform the jump, so long as both feet remain on the ground. The arms can be used to help propel the body upward and one arm is used to stretch for the highest points. As you crouch down for the jump, move your arms down and behind your buttocks. As you jump upward, fling your arms upward. The movement of the arms increases the upward force of the jump and also maximizes the height at which the jump is measured.

Training Tips

The vertical jump ultimately measures the explosive power of your legs. As the preliminary move in a vertical jump is a squat, it makes sense to practice squats as part of your training. Look at the squats section on pages 156–57 to see the variations on squats that you can do, including squats with weights, such as dumbbells. Once your body can perform sets of squats with weights its explosive upward power will be greatly increased.

Other training exercises include:
- **Tuck jump:** Jump upward, pulling your knees toward your chest before landing
- **Box jump:** Jump up onto a secure box or fixed platform 18in (45cm) high
- **Burpee:** Get down on your haunches, then stand up to do a tuck jump

CLIMBING A ROPE MARINE STYLE

Rope climbing is a very testing exercise and it is considered to be vital in training for the US and Royal Marines, as well as for special forces such as US Navy SEALs. It tests upper-body strength (mainly the arms) but, as with rock climbing, the legs play a vital role. To maximize the effect of the legs, to increase speed, and to minimize arm fatigue, correct technique is essential. You can support yourself on a rope with your arms for a short while, but for longer duration you will need to rely on your legs.

1. Wear boots or sturdy shoes.

2. Grip the rope as high as you can with your hands.

3. Let the rope pass between your legs, around your knee and calf, and back between the instep of the boots.

4. Clamp your feet together, trapping the rope.

5. Push down on your feet and on the rope and simultaneously pull up with your arms in a coordinated movement.

6. Gripping the rope with your hands in the new position, loosen the grip with your feet by raising the top boot off the rope and slide both feet upward, keeping the rope in the same position around the calf.

7. Lock the rope again with your feet and repeat.

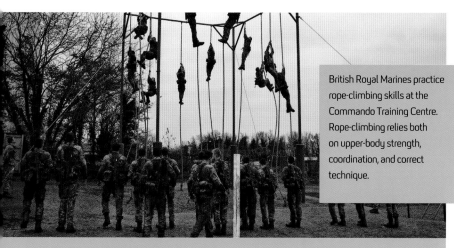

British Royal Marines practice rope-climbing skills at the Commando Training Centre. Rope-climbing relies both on upper-body strength, coordination, and correct technique.

US Navy SEAL rope-climbing technique

The US Navy SEALs sometimes use an alternative rope-climbing technique to that used by the Marines.

1. Reach up and pull yourself up on the rope.

2. Bend your outside leg (the leg furthest away from the rope) and place the top of your foot on the outside of the rope.

3. Simultaneously, use the outside of one foot to push the rope over your other foot and push it down.

4. The rope then passes under one foot and over the other foot. Your feet should now close together to lock the rope.

5. To move upward, slide both feet upward, allowing the rope to pass over one foot and under the other. Then press down and lock to create a base for further upward movement.

THE BLEEP TEST

The bleep test, also known as the beep test, the shuttle run, and the multi-stage fitness test, involves running between two points on a 22yd (20m) track, keeping up with a series of beeps on a preset recording. The formal description of the test is "progressive aerobic cardiovascular endurance test." The test is especially useful for sports that require short bursts of speed, such as rugby, football, netball, and tennis, and also for military training.

The Rules

The test progresses through a series of levels, becoming faster each time, testing the athlete's ability to keep pace. There are up to 21 levels, which increase the speed by 0.3 mph (0.5kph) from a base level of 5.3mph (8.5kph) as the level rises. To signal the change of level there are three quick beeps.

If the contestant does not reach the line before the beep sounds, they are given a warning. They must continue to run to the line and then catch up before two more beeps sound. If the contestant cannot reach the line before the beep for two consecutive ends, then that is marked as their level and they finish the test.

Although the bleep test is in many respects a scientific test of maximum fitness and VO_2 max, it can be affected by environmental factors as well as by technique. Environmental factors may include weather conditions and running surface, while technique may include running efficiency, turning, and familiarity.

MUSCLES WORKED

- ☑ *Gastrocnemius/soleus (calf muscles)*
- ☑ *Tibialis anterior (shin)*
- ☑ *Semitendinosus, semimembranosus, and biceps femoris (hamstrings/back of thigh)*
- ☑ *Quadriceps (front of thigh)*
- ☑ *Gluteus maximus (buttocks)*
- ☑ *Adductors and abductors (inner and outer thigh)*
- ☑ *Rectus abdominus, obliques, erector spinea, and transverse abdominus (core muscles)*
- ☑ *Anterior deltoid (shoulders)*
- ☑ *Latissimus dorsi and posterior deltoid (back)*

Variants

Different military services require different levels in the bleep test. Not surprisingly, the standards for elite and special forces are significantly higher than those for regular armed forces entry. In the Australian Army, the entry requirement is 7.5, equivalent to 56 shuttles or a total of 1,225yd (1,120m) in 6:30 minutes. In the elite regiments of the British Armed Forces, the Royal Marines and the Parachute Regiment, the minimum score is 13.

Strategies

Although the whole point of the bleep test is to test your aerobic fitness, which you can develop in activities such as running or team sports, you can improve your chances of doing well by using the right technique. When you reach the line, ensure you place only one foot over the line and turn efficiently so that you don't waste time and energy taking a wide-arc turn. Make sure you push away strongly after the turn so that you get quickly back up to speed. When the level moves up, focus on getting into the new level fast and keeping it up. Keep your breathing smooth. Lean forward slightly and keep your body and arms relaxed.

Training Tips

The bleep test is about aerobic fitness, endurance, speed, agility, and running. To train for the bleep test you need to cover all of these bases. Go for long, slow endurance runs to build your base aerobic fitness and endurance. To improve your ability to accelerate over short distances, try fartlek (speed play, see page 30), which involves running at a higher pace for short distances in the context of a longer run.

WALKING/ MARCHING

Walking is the most basic and natural exercise. Early hunter-gatherers did not go jogging; they walked and only ran when they needed to, such as making the final chase on prey or running away from danger. Military personnel only run in extreme situations, to get under cover or maneuver in a firefight. Otherwise, military personnel mostly walk, often carrying weight, such as a pack and/or webbing.

Variants

Walking is an excellent warm-up routine. If you are planning to do some weight training, go for a walk beforehand (walk the dog or buy a newspaper) to give your body time to adjust and for your spine to be invigorated.

In a real military situation, troops may be required to get to their destination in the shortest possible time on foot carrying all of their equipment. This would normally include:

- A pack weighing about 45lb (20kg)
- Webbing/load-bearing equipment (LBE)

- A weapon weighing about 8lb (3.6kg) They would also be wearing full battle fatigues and military boots.

Strategies

Because walking is such a basic human activity, little thought, if any, is usually given to how to walk efficiently. But following a good walking technique can help to avoid injury and optimize your efficiency. You should walk through your foot by placing your heel gently but firmly on the ground and rolling through the midfoot before pushing off with the ball of your foot. (NB: This is different from the running footfall, where your

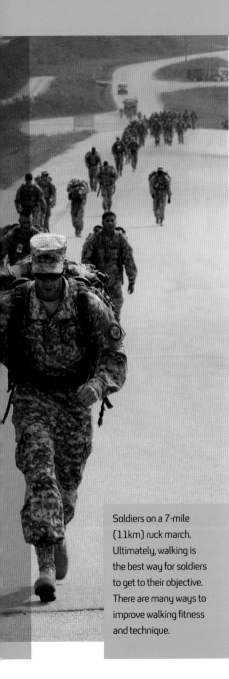

Soldiers on a 7-mile (11km) ruck march. Ultimately, walking is the best way for soldiers to get to their objective. There are many ways to improve walking fitness and technique.

body will be leaning forward and where it is recommended that you land on your midfoot.) Remember to walk tall, holding your ribcage up and keeping your midriff firm. The US Special Forces guidelines on walking are as follows:

- Keep the weight of your body directly over your feet.
- Keep the sole of your boot/shoe flat on the ground at all times.
- Take small steps at an even pace.
- On cross-country walks, go around obstacles or step over them; never step on them.
- When walking up steep slopes, use a zigzag pattern to reduce the impact of the gradient.
- When descending steep slopes, keep your back straight and your knees bent to soak up the shock. Dig your heels in.
- Practice walking as fast as you can with a backpack but do not run with a backpack as it may cause an injury.
- Keep going at a fast pace for 6 to 8 miles (9.7–12.9km) and then take a short break (about 5 minutes).

Wear supportive walking shoes that encourage the rolling motion of the foot. For military training you will be expected to wear boots so it is a good idea to select a comfortable pair and to learn to run in them. Buy good quality walking socks. For winter walking these should

MUSCLES WORKED

- ☑ *Gastrocnemius/soleus (calf muscles)*
- ☑ *Tibialis anterior (shin)*
- ☑ *Semitendinosus, semimembranosus, and biceps femoris (hamstrings/back of thigh)*
- ☑ *Quadriceps (front of thigh)*
- ☑ *Gluteus maximus (buttocks)*
- ☑ *Adductors and abductors (inner and outer thigh)*
- ☑ *Rectus abdominus, obliques, erector spinea, and transverse abdominus (core muscles)*
- ☑ *Anterior deltoid (shoulders)*
- ☑ *Latissimus dorsi and posterior deltoid (back)*

walking these should be thicker and may contain wool such as Merino for warmth and minimum moisture retention. For summer, wear thinner socks so that your feet do not get too hot. Consider wearing two pairs of socks: one thin inner pair and a thicker outer pair. This may reduce the occurrence of blisters. If you are wearing military boots, consider adding an impact absorbing insole.

When you are walking medium to long distances, adapt your clothing according to the weather conditions and according to the increase in body heat as you

exercise. It is best to wear layers that can be removed when necessary and put in a backpack. Take water to rehydrate if you are out for a long period.

Training Tips

If you are at the beginning of a fitness building regime, walking, along with strength training, is one of the best ways of building bone mass. It also has the advantage that it does not place a strain on the body in the same way that running does, for example. Military walking requires you to have aerobic fitness and helps you to develop it further. It also builds endurance, physical and mental. To prepare for the walking aspects of military training, you should start walking first without weights, gradually increasing your distance, and then building up the weight you carry.

Bear in mind that as you carry heavier weights on your back, you will need to wear shoes or boots that are supportive enough to take the extra weight. To begin with, carry a pack that is about 10 percent of your body weight and build it up from there. As an alternative to practicing marches with a backpack, you can do squats (for example, perform 5 sets of 100 repetitions).

When on a military-style walk or march, the aim is to not only get from A to B as quickly and efficiently as possible—you then need to be able to function and do your job at the other end (which may mean building a shelter, digging a trench, patrolling or, yes, fighting an enemy). Sorry, no hot shower or a bath after a real military walk…!

UK Royal Marines speed march

Here is an example of a military march that you could attempt in order to test yourself. Requirements:

- About 21lb (14kg) personal load carrying equipment
- Combat clothing and boots
- **Weapon:** about 9lb (4kg)
- **Distance:** 4 miles (6.4km)
- **Completion time:** Under 40 minutes

The march is conducted over varied, challenging terrain. Remember to stay well hydrated with water throughout the march.

WALKING HEALTHY

The recommended amount of walking each day for health is 30 minutes per day. Walking has a huge range of benefits:

— It reduces the risk of catching infections and diseases.
— It keeps the body toned and weight down.
— It boosts the levels of Vitamin D in your body.
— It strengthens your heart and boosts circulation.
— It improves muscle endurance.
— Walking is low impact exercise and therefore has much less risk of injury than other higher impact forms of exercise such as running.
— Military-style walking can be as beneficial as jogging for burning calories.
— Walking is more beneficial for the spine than running as it puts less pressure on the discs in your spine.
— Regular walking pumps vitamins and minerals through the spine.
— It helps to improve sleep and brain function.

RUNNING

If you are taking up running for the first time as part of a military fitness training program, it is a good idea to learn good habits from the start. If you are a more experienced runner, you can also improve your technique if necessary. Posture, foot strike, and cadence (the number of steps you take in a given time) are some of the areas worth paying attention to when working on your running technique.

Variants

As there are different types of running tests, you need to train to cover both long distance and sprinting. For example, a running test may be a 87yd (80m) sprint, a 22yd (20m) shuttle run, or a 1.5-mile (2.4km) run. The good news is that any kind of running training will help you to achieve your goals. Long slow distance (LSD) will build up a base of endurance and aerobic fitness. On this basis, you can build your speed running, which may include fartlek (speed play) within a longer run, a pace run (running at just below VO$_2$ max throughout your run) and 437yd (400m), 219yd (200m), and 110yd (100m) sprint training. Resistance running (up hills) will help to improve strength (try running uphill with a long pace as if you were on the flat) and trail running will improve your body's ability to maintain balance on uneven terrain.

Strategies

Posture

Bad posture and incorrect running form can lead to injuries, as well as making your running less efficient. Typical signs of bad running form are a slouching posture, bending from the waist, over-striding, and heel-striking. The ideal running form is to keep the body straight (imagine a line running through your upper thigh, up your back, and into your neck), a slightly forward leaning posture, and a midfoot strike on the ground.

In order to optimize your posture before you start to run, stand straight, lock your fingers together, and raise your arms above your head, pushing upward to elongate your spine. Then relax your arms at your side, holding them at a 90-degree angle, and keeping both arms and shoulders relaxed.

When you are running, keep your arms moving in an easy but controlled movement and do not let your arms cross the center line of your body.

Foot strike

If you run barefoot, on a beach for example, you will notice that you strike the ground with the midsection of the foot. This is a natural way for the body to absorb the shock of landing.

If you land on your heel bone, the shock is communicated straight up to your back. Although cushioned running shoes absorb much of the shock of a heel strike, the principle remains the same when running in shoes.

BAD POSTURE AND INCORRECT RUNNING FORM CAN LEAD TO INJURIES AND MAKE YOUR RUNNING LESS EFFICIENT

If you land on your midfoot, the foot rolls more naturally through the foot strike and forward roll, eliminating the jarring and braking effect of a heel strike. It may take some time to accustom yourself to midfoot running. Try running on the spot to feel the contact of the midfoot on the ground. Also, consider using lower profile running shoes that will help you to place more emphasis on the midfoot strike and help to improve your running stance.

Before you start your run, lean forward slightly at the ankles and let your body move naturally into the running motion with the aid of gravity.

Training Tips

Aim for 180 steps per minute or three steps every second. As you learn to do this, you will find that you will be less

YOU NEED A SOLID FOUNDATION OF MEDIUM- TO LONG-DISTANCE RUNNING BEFORE YOU WORK ON YOUR SPEED

likely to push your legs out ahead of you in long strides. Remember that the military physical fitness test is about time over a set distance—usually 1.5 or 2 miles (2.4–3.2km), but also 3 miles (4.8km) for elite and special forces entry. You need to first build your overall running fitness and then focus on building your pace.

One of the best ways of increasing pace over a period of time is interval training. First you need to establish a base time so that you know what your goals are. If you want to achieve the US Marine Corps running time, for example, you need to be able to run:

- ½ mile (0.2km) in 3 minutes
- ¼ mile (0.4km) in 90 seconds
- ⅛ mile (0.8km) in 45 seconds

As you attempt to achieve each of these times, give yourself plenty of time for a cool-down in between. So, walk for ¼ mile (0.4km) to recover if you are at an early stage in your training. If you are fit, you may want to jog instead. Set your goal time and repeat it three or four times. For example:

- Run ½ mile (0.8km) at your maximum goal pace
- Then walk or jog for ¼ mile (0.4km)
- Repeat this between four and six times
- Run ¼ mile (0.4km) at maximum goal pace
- Then walk or jog for ⅛ mile (0.2km)
- Repeat this between four and six times
- Run ⅛ mile (0.2km) at goal pace
- Then walk or jog for 100yd (91m)

Spread this workout so that you repeat it twice a week. In between, do some longer runs of between 3 and 5 miles (4.8–8km), to work on your underlying fitness.

Building a foundation

It is a basic and accepted principle among professional runners that you need a solid foundation of medium to long-distance running before you work on your speed. As a minimum, you should consider running between 20 and 25 miles (32–40km) per week.

Workout 1

- Run 1 mile (1.6km) at an easy pace
- Repeat this between eight and ten times
- Run ¼ mile (0.4km) at 10–20 seconds under your current mile pace
- To recover, walk or slow jog for a minute

Workout 2

- Run 1 mile (1.6km) at an easy pace
- Repeat this five times
- Run ½-mile (0.8km) stretches at 10 seconds under your current mile pace
- Walk or jog slowly for 2 minutes

Workout 3

- Run 1 mile (1.6km) at an easy pace
- Then run 1 mile (1.6km) at 10 seconds above your current mile pace
- Jog for 2 minutes at a slow pace
- Run 1 mile (1.6km) at your current mile pace
- Walk or jog slowly for 2 minutes
- Then run 1 mile (1.6km) at 10 seconds faster than your current mile pace
- Jog for about 5 minutes
- Then stretch

Workout 4

- Run for 5 minutes as a warm-up and then stretch
- Then run for 3 minutes, incorporating 1-minute sprints followed by 1-minute slow jogs

SWIMMING

Similar rules apply in swimming as to running. You need to build a base of long slow distance (LSD) training to build endurance, alongside your high-intensity workouts, which are designed to increase your speed. Swimming and running can complement each other. As the water provides overall support for the body, swimming can help to tone muscles and release tension.

Variants

Aside from the front crawl and breaststroke, if you are interested in training to high military fitness standards you might also want to master the combat sidestroke. It was developed to enable special forces personnel, and marines in particular, to travel efficiently through the water while maintaining a low profile. The swimmer always keeps their hands below the surface so as not to break water and attract attention. The combat sidestroke should help you to swim long distances with the least amount of energy and also to swim through the surf zone.

To start the stroke, begin on your stomach and then move onto your side and then back onto your stomach.

1. Place your body in the streamline position, with your body flat on your stomach, your arms out ahead, your face pointing downward, and your legs straight out behind you.
2. Pull your left arm downward, keeping your right arm straight.
3. Turn your body toward the right, so that the left shoulder rises to the surface and the body is sideways.
4. Keep pushing your stroke arm down toward your thigh, while your head comes out of the water.

5. Once the stroke is complete, move the hand back up the body, while pulling downward with the other arm.

6. As your two hands meet near your upper chest, move your knee forward for the scissor kick, which will help to take you back to the streamline position. The scissor kick involves pushing the water with both the top of the bottom foot and the bottom of the top foot.

7. Move both hands forward together ahead of you to the original streamline position.

Flutter kick

Use the flutter kick with or without flippers by moving the legs at the hips. Your legs should be straight out behind you without being rigid and with a slight bend in the knee. Your toes should also be pointed out behind you, though your ankle should remain flexible. If you are performing the flutter kick without flippers, your leg movement from the hips should be faster due to the reduced surface area, whereas with fins the movement will be slower and deeper.

Strategies

One of the most important things to get right when swimming with any stroke is breathing. It is particularly important for the front crawl. You need to take in sufficient air, while also timing it correctly so that it does not interfere with your stroke. If you don't take in enough air, you will soon start to build up a deficit and come to a grinding halt. The more you swim, the more you will train your lungs to expand and cope with shorter intakes of breath.

There are different swimming strategies for different strokes and there is not enough room to discuss them all in detail here. Overall strategies include:

- **Streamlining:** Keep your head in line with your body as much as possible.
- **Regularity:** Although much of the focus is on your arm stroke, always remember to maintain a steady kick.
- **Turning:** Practice your turning, as you can lose valuable time on a bad or slow turn, which will compromise all your other hard work and training.
- **Catch:** Pay attention to the shape of your hand in the water and the movement of your arms through the water. Your hand should be flat and slightly cupped, with the fingers closed.
- **Recovery:** Move your arms back into position for the next stroke as soon as possible.

Breaststroke

- Keep your body level and on the surface of the water in order to minimize drag.
- Keep your shoulders in line and your hips flat on the water.
- The most complex movement in the breaststroke is the leg movement. Practice the froglike leg movements while holding on to the side of the pool until they become natural. The movements of both legs must mirror each other.
- Take a long stretch between each stroke, streamlining your body so that you move efficiently through the water.
- Make sure you can see your hands at all times when performing an arm stroke.
- Make sure your legs and arms stay on the water at all times.
- Breathe in as you finish the circle stroke with your arms.

Front crawl

Breathing: This is the priority with the crawl because there is no point having the perfect stroke if you are spluttering and gasping for breath halfway across the pool. Turn your head as smoothly as possible so that one side of your face is on the surface of the water.

TAKE TIME TO PRACTICE YOUR TECHNIQUE WITH SLOW SWIMS

Blow out strongly in the water before you turn your head to take a breath. After taking your breath, turn your head back into the water. Work out which breathing routine suits you best, e.g., after either two, three, or four strokes.

Posture: Keep your body close to the surface. Your hips and legs should be on the same level as your shoulders.

Legs: Your legs play a vital role in keeping you straight, so keep kicking regularly.

Hands: Place your hand sideways into the water, thumb first.

Arms: Keep driving your arm under the water until your hand reaches the top of your leg.

Recovery: When taking your arm out of the water, lift your elbow out first so that it is pointing toward the sky.

Training Tips

With all of the above, take time to practice your technique with slow swims, which will allow you to concentrate on your movements and develop good practice. Make sure you warm up and cool down properly before and after swimming. Start with a gentle 5-minute swim. Swimming uses most of the major muscle groups so pay attention to stretches on your calves, quadriceps, hamstrings, pectorals, trapezius, triceps, deltoids, and abdominals. Hold each stretch for up to 15 seconds. For a cool-down, swim about five laps, getting slower each lap. Use a variety of strokes. Use a kickboard to swim slowly for another two laps, using flutter kicks and breaststroke kicks. Hang on to the side of the pool and bring your knees up to your chest before bending your head gently forward. Stand straight and raise yourself up onto your toes. Raise your arms above your head and cross your elbows before turning gently from left to right. Have a warm shower!

Workouts may include:

5 × 55yd (50m) freestyle (20 seconds rest between each)

5 × 110yd (100m) sprints (any stroke; a minute rest between each)

Kickboard

5 × 55–110yd (50–100m) sprint (flutter kicks)

5 × 55–110yd (50–100m) sprint (breaststroke kicks)

Swim with flippers for up to 30 minutes.

Try mixing in other training on the side of the pool, such as push-ups and sit-ups. Use any training equipment available for more strength training exercises.

OBSTACLE COURSE

The obstacle course is a standard part of military training as it replicates the kinds of obstacles military personnel might encounter in the course of active duty. It tests the full range of military fitness and mental attitude, including endurance, determination, balance, lower- and upper-body strength, and teamwork (some obstacles, such as the 8ft/2.5m wall, are best surmounted with the help of teammates).

Variants

There is a huge variety of military obstacle courses. Some civilian obstacle courses are modeled on military courses and these are increasing in popularity. Depending on the units for which they are intended or the type of operations that they are designed to assess suitability for, military obstacle courses may place emphasis on particular areas. "Nasty Nick" at Camp Marshall, Fort Bragg, Carolina, includes a giant upright ladder as well as rope climbs up to 30ft (9m). This is where US Army Special Forces do their basic training. At Hindersnisstreike in Germany there is a course that places emphasis on overcoming fear of heights. Recruits must cross a cable at height while holding on to a parallel cable and also climb a high wall. At Fort Benning, the recruits must negotiate smaller obstacles, including hurdle bars and low walls at speed, before coming upon the inevitable rope climb. This form of course simulates the sort of obstacles that units such as the US Marines would expect to meet in an assault. Many courses are based on wooden structures and have an "outdoors" theme. Some are designed to simulate urban environments, where surfaces are smooth and hard.

An obstacle course for general training may include some of the following:

Steps

A set of parallel crossbars of increasing height.

Technique: Keep your eyes on the bars so that you don't miss your step. Hit each bar with your midfoot to avoid slipping. Keep up your momentum, leaning slightly forward from your ankles.

Double ditch

Leap across a ditch onto a raised area and then jump across another ditch.

Technique: Keep your momentum as you make the jump and try to use the latent momentum to make the second jump.

Crawl

Crawl across an area under low wires.

Technique: You will need to use both your forearms and your lower legs to push yourself forward. Use the sides of your boots to get as much traction as you can on the ground.

Wall (low)

This could be a 6ft (1.8m) wall that you should climb over without assistance.

Technique: A confident approach is the key to getting over a wall. One method is to jump up and get both forearms on top of the wall and then hook one leg over to pull up your body with leg strength.

Dry ditch

Leap across a sandy area onto a slope on the other side.

Technique: The key here is a confident approach with good forward momentum. Make sure you land with your foot flat on the sloped surface and maintain the momentum to power yourself up.

Ramp

Run up and jump down the other side.

Technique: Momentum is vital and you should make sure that you keep your feet flat on the surface, which may well be wet and slippery.

Rope swing

Run up to a platform, grasp a rope, and swing across a ditch (often filled with water) to land on a ramp on the other side. If you fall in the water, you have to attempt it again with wet clothes.

Technique: Grasp the rope high and give yourself plenty of momentum for the push-off. If you grab the rope too low, you will swing too low to get onto the ramp on the other side. Quickly look at the other side to assess the effort required to get there, and then focus on the rope.

MUSCLES WORKED

An obstacle course tests every muscle you have and even ones you didn't know you had before you started. Many muscles have been described in this section but perhaps one set of muscles you will notice the need for in an obstacle course is your hands, especially when grabbing ropes or hanging on monkey bars. That hand grip could make the difference between staying dry or landing in muddy water.

High wall

The high wall will probably require a team effort.

Technique: Help one teammate onto the wall. This teammate can then turn, with their legs over the other side, and reach down to haul you up.

Beam balance

Climb up a railing and then balance on beams taking you to the other side where you will find ropes to climb down.

Technique: The beam balance is all about confidence and focus. Place each foot pointing outward on the beam and keep your midfoot on the beam. Keep your arms outstretched for balance. Try to maintain your forward momentum, without rushing.

Treble stride ditch

Leap up to and across beams at right angles to your approach.

Technique: Keep an adequate forward momentum and keep your eyes on the beams. Land on each beam with your midfoot and keep your weight balanced over your feet so that you don't slip.

Overhand traverse "monkey bars"

Jump up to a series of ladder bars and swing yourself across a ditch, using arm strength and forward momentum.

Technique: Momentum is key to the monkey bars. Use your legs and lower body to swing yourself forward as you grab for each bar.

Stepping stones

This can be an arrangement of stones or small pillars at varying heights. On some obstacle courses, some stones can be "floating" in water while others are solid.

Technique: Keep your eyes on the stones and keep up your momentum. Keep your feet flat on the stones or pillars and don't push off too hard. Keep your weight balanced over your feet.

Scramble net

Scramble to the top of the net where you climb over a bar and then scramble down the other side.

Technique: When you reach the top bar, make sure you keep one hand on the rope on the nearside as you reach over and grasp the rope on the far side. Then swing your legs over. Once you have found a footing for both feet, bring your hand over from the first side and grasp the rope on the second side.

Tube crawl

Crawl through tubes until you get to the other side. There will be plenty of muddy water inside!

Technique: Use your elbows and feet to push on the walls of the tunnel to push yourself through.

Burma bridge

Climb up ladder bars then crawl across a rope bridge to the other side before jumping down.

Technique: You will need to keep your momentum up on the rope bridge by using both hands and feet to pull and push yourself forward. Try to avoid sticking arms or hands through the gaps in the net.

Swinging duckboards

Walk across one of the duckboards, which is suspended on ropes or chains and liable to move under your feet. You need to maintain your balance.

Technique: Keep your momentum up and your feet flat on the duckboards. Keep your arms out for balance and your weight balanced over your feet.

Climbing ropes

Climb a rope to the required height and then let yourself down under control before running on to finish the course.

Technique: Legs are vital in rope climbing, even though it may look like it depends on the arms. Make sure you can get a grip on the rope with your feet and legs.

Training Tips

When practicing for obstacle courses, find a local course that is open to civilians or use natural or manmade obstacles. A military obstacle course is normally run in boots and combat trousers. Tough trousers and a long-sleeve top will help to protect your legs and arms. Beware when practicing in winter or after rain that any obstacles made from wood will be very slippery and potentially dangerous.

ERGOMETER

Ergometers are machines, in the form of exercise bicycles, treadmills, or static rowing machines, that can provide accurate indications of endurance and VO_2 max (the maximum amount of oxygen in milliliters that you can use during intensive workout). Some military testers use ergometers as part of their fitness tests, while others recommend them as part of your build-up training plan.

Variants

The bicycle ergometer is sometimes used to test endurance and VO_2 max (aerobic efficiency), particularly of the legs, in a static environment. The work intensity can be regulated by changing the resistance and cycling rate. Bicycle ergometers can either be mechanically or electronically braked. If it is a mechanically braked ergometer, a specified cycling rate must be maintained in order to keep the work rate constant. An electronically braked ergometer will automatically adjust the internal resistance to maintain a specified work rate according to the cycling rate.

The work rate should be adjusted in increments, either automatically or manually. Like any standard bicycle, the cycle ergometer has handlebars and an adjustable seat. The pedals should include grips for optimum traction.

A treadmill is a form of ergometer sometimes used in military tests (e.g. UK Royal Navy). The advantage of the treadmill from the military tester's perspective is that it offers a standardized method of testing without the variations of terrain, temperature, and weather conditions encountered outdoors.

Bicycle

To make the most of the test, ensure that the seat is set at the correct height so that your knee is slightly flexed at full extension, while allowing you to use the full power of your leg.

You cannot expect to do well in a test without previous exercise/a warm-up. You should also practice on an ergometer in your local gym. The other obvious way to train yourself is on a road bike. The Wingate Test Protocol is often used as a standard test. It is used to test peak anaerobic power, anaerobic fatigue, and total anaerobic capacity.

Wingate Test Protocol

Warm-up	5 minutes	Low-intensity cycling mixed with 4 or 5 sprints of 4 seconds
Recovery	2–5 minutes	Slow cycling
Max acceleration	15 seconds	Cycle for 10 seconds at a third of the prescribed force setting, then build to prescribed force within 5 seconds
Wingate test	30 seconds	Cycle for 10 seconds at a third of the prescribed force setting, then build to prescribed force setting within 5 seconds
Cool down	1–2 minutes	Cycling at low to moderate aerobic power

REAL RUNNING AND CYCLING ARE GOOD TRAINING FOR THE TREADMILL AND THE CYCLE ERGOMETER

Treadmill

When using a treadmill, ensure that it is set to a pace that you can keep up with. If you have to keep grabbing the bars, it usually means that you are going too fast. Whenever you use a treadmill, the same rules apply for warm-ups and cool-downs as when you are running outside. To warm up for a distance run on a treadmill try the following schedule:

- Warm up for 3 minutes
- Easy run for 2 minutes
- Walk for 1 minute
- Repeat three times

A treadmill can, to some extent, act as a substitute for a coach. As a reminder, most military fitness tests include some form of running, which could be either a 1.5-mile (2.4km) or 3-mile (4.8km) run.

Rowing machine

The rowing machine is a very useful training aid as it helps significantly with cardio respiratory fitness, while also working up to 70 percent of the muscles in the body. As a low impact activity, rowing works well as part of an overall training plan, allowing you to take the strain off legs that have become tired or injured from running, for example. Rowing machines of course provide excellent training for those involved in competition rowing on water.

Training Tips

Some treadmills can be set to military fitness standards. This means that the treadmill will provide you with the results according to the test requirements. Feed in the required information, such as your age, sex, and so on, and the machine will make the necessary calculations against your performance.

Make sure you are aware of the particular settings that suit you. When on a cycle ergometer, pay particular attention to your leg length so that you get maximum power. Remember that real running and real cycling are good training for the treadmill and the cycle ergometer.

The technology built into ergometers such as this treadmill can provide useful information about your fitness levels and overall progress.

MUSCLES WORKED

Cycle ergometer
☑ Gluteus maximus (buttocks)
☑ Quadriceps (front of thigh)
☑ Semimembranosus (hamstrings)
☑ Soleus (inner calf)
☑ Gastrocnemius (outer calf)

Treadmill
☑ Quadriceps (front of thigh)
☑ Hamstrings (back of thigh)
☑ Soleus (inner calf)
☑ Gastrocnemius (outer calf)
☑ Gluteus maximus (buttocks)
☑ Hip flexors/extenders
☑ Biceps brachii (top of upper arm)
☑ Rectus abdominis (abdominals)
☑ Intercostales externii (external rib muscles)
☑ Intercostales interni (internal rib muscles)

Rowing machine
☑ Quadriceps (front of thigh)
☑ Hamstrings (back of thigh)
☑ Gluteus maximus (buttocks)
☑ Rectus abdominis (abs/abdominal muscles)
☑ Transverse abdominis (abdominal muscle)
☑ Obliques (side abdominals)
☑ Erector spinae (back)
☑ Upper trapezius (shoulder blade)
☑ Rhomboids (upper back)
☑ Latissimus dorsi (mid-back)
☑ Triceps (back upper arm)
☑ Anterior deltoids (back of shoulder)
☑ Iliopsoas (hip)

RESOURCES

Military websites

Australian Defence Force
http://www.defencejobs.gov.au/fitness/

ADF Recruitment Centre
http://www.defencejobs.gov.au/
recruitmentCentre/canIJoin/healthAndFitness/

Belgian Armed Forces
http://www.rma.ac.be/fr/rma-sport-
evaluation-fr.html

British Army
http://www.army.mod.uk/infantry/regiments/
parachute/26245.aspx
http://www.army.mod.uk/join/Getting-
yourself-ready.aspx

Canadian Armed Forces
http://www.forces.ca/en/page/training-
90#tab2
http://www.forces.gc.ca/en/index.page

Danish Defence Force
http://forsvaret.dk/FKO/eng/Pages/default.
aspx
http://forsvaret.dk/JGK/Pages/default.aspx

Jagerkorpset
http://forsvaret.dk/jgk/Pages/default.aspx

Dutch Korps Mariniers
http://korpsmariniers.com/

Finnish Defence Forces
http://www.puolustusvoimat.fi/en/

French Army recruitment
http://www.recrutement.terre.defense.gouv.fr/

French Foreign Legion
http://www.legion-etrangere.
com/?block=19&titre=le-portail

Kampfschwimmer
http://www.kampfschwimmer.de/

Indian Air Force
http://indianairforce.nic.in/?id=3

Irish Defense Forces
http://www.military.ie/en/home/

The Netherlands Ministry of Defence
http://www.defensie.nl/english

New Zealand Defense Force
Force Fit
http://www.defencecareers.mil.nz/force-fit

NZDF Fitness Requirements
http://www.defencecareers.mil.nz/army/
joining-up/fitness-requirements

New Zealand Special Air Service (NZSAS)
http://www.army.mil.nz/about-us/who-we-
are/nzsas/default.htm

Norwegian Armed Forces
http://mil.no/Pages/default.aspx

Royal Australian Navy
http://www.navy.gov.au/

RAN Recruit school fitness
http://www.navy.gov.au/join-navy/recruit-school/fitness

Royal Marines (United Kingdom)
http://www.royalnavy.mod.uk/careers/royal-marines

Royal Marines training tool
http://www.royalnavy.mod.uk/custom/navy/trainingtool.html

Royal Navy (United Kingdom)
https://pdevportal.co.uk/physical_training

Spanish Armed Forces
http://www.reclutamiento.defensa.gob.es/suboficiales/como_ingresar/pruebas.htm

Swedish Armed Forces
http://www.forsvarsmakten.se/en/

Swiss Armed Forces
http://www.vtg.admin.ch/internet/vtg/en/home.html

US Navy
http://www.navy.mil/

US Navy Fitness and Deployed Forces Support
http://www.navyfitness.org/

US Marine Corps
http://www.marines.com/home

Other websites

American College of Sport Medicine
http://www.acsm.org/

Good Form Running
http://www.goodformrunning.com/

Military Fitness website
http://www.military.com/military-fitness

Books

Dale, Patrick. *Military Fitness*. London, UK: Robert Hale, 2012.

Weale, Adrian. *Fighting Fit*. London, UK: Orion, 1995.

INDEX

CREDITS